*Your Guide to a Longer
and Healthier Life*

LifeGuide
Volume 1

Second Edition

*How to Avoid The Illnesses
Created by Modern Man*

David Perlmutter, M.D.

Board Certified Practicing Neurologist

LifeGuide Press
Publishers
Naples, Florida
USA

LifeGuide Press

Publishers

Naples, Florida

USA

ISBN 0-9635874-0-4

The views and opinions expressed herein are solely those of the author and are expressed for the purpose of stimulating thought and discussion. This book should not be construed as specific medical advice to any reader or recipient of the information.

Opinions and views presented herein are not intended and should not be construed as creating any type of physician-patient relationship. Readers should consult their personal physicians with specific questions regarding any of the subject matter presented herein.

Acknowledgments

I would like to thank the following special people for their support and inspiration: my friend and partner in Naples Neurological Associates, William D. Ertag, M.D., for his continuing commitment to medicine and confidence in my work, as well as fellow neurologist, John D. Campbell, and the entire staff at Naples Neurological Associates. In addition, special thanks to Donna and Corbin Wyant, who made my newspaper column a reality, Heather Burch of the Pathfinders Institute and the Rev. Dick Smith for their love and continuing encouragement, Bruce and Cheryl Scheiner of the law firm Associates and Bruce L. Scheiner, for their generous support of the *LifeGuide* television series, and two special people, Matt Crist and Bill Pogue.

The *LifeGuide* Foundation

The LifeGuide Foundation is a non-profit organization with the goal of providing to the public health-related information which is critically under-utilized in the Western medical world.

Ultimately, this foundation will serve as the vehicle for creating the *LifeGuide Clinic*, a facility which will utilize the holistic perspective in disease prevention and treatment. In this clinic, a wide range of complementary modalities will serve the body, mind and spirit of each individual patient.

The *LifeGuide Clinic* will represent not an *alternative* choice, standing apart from modern Western medicine. Rather, our approach will be truly *complementary* —recognizing the achievements of modern Western medical technology that are useful, and incorporating them into a total treatment plan. This truly holistic approach will honor the body's natural healing abilities; not only in treating disease, but in maintaining good health.

The goals of the *LifeGuide Clinic* will be achieved through funds generated by the sale of this book, together with other fund-raising efforts and charitable contributions from individuals and corporations.

We thank you for your support. For more information about The *LifeGuide Foundation*, write to us at:

The *LifeGuide* Foundation

720 Goodlette Road, North, Suite 203-L

Naples, Florida 33940

I wish to thank my wife, Leize, who has lovingly and persistently guided me in my exploration of alternative health choices; my father, whose professionalism and dedication to the art of medicine continues to serve as an inspiration; my mother, whose wart removal technique (using a potato under the light of a full moon) provided my first exposure to non-mainstream medicine; and Austin and Reisha, beacons of the future. In addition, this book would not have come into fruition had it not been for Karen Lee; especially her persistence in helping me recognize the importance of getting this message out and my ability to do so.

Table of Contents

Introduction

What is a doctor? This word, derived from Latin, doesn't mean healer, it means teacher—one who gives people the knowledge they need to facilitate their own healing processes and achieve a state of well-being.

This book was created to help you deal with a variety of medical problems, reduce or eliminate your dependence upon pharmaceutical drugs, and maintain optimum health.

LifeGuide explores alternatives—alternatives to the contemporary emphasis on drugs as "magic bullets" for curing diseases. It is about taking responsibility for your own well-being by examining the habits, diets and addictions that have become so common in Western society. It's about encouraging your physician to appreciate you as a whole person as opposed to another case a particular illness.

In ancient China, the physician was rewarded only when the people of his village experienced health. His role was to maintain health and harmony, rather than fighting disease. Instead of fostering health and harmony, the role of today's physician is to wage war against the various illnesses our modern society has created. Illness today is treated reflexively, as doctors attack disease with ferocious determination, all but ignoring the patient. Too often the immediate response to controlling disease is to prescribe whichever drug is being best promoted.

Those involved in alternative medicine know that uncovering the mysteries of a health problem takes a little more work for both the patient and physician. It takes dedication on the patient's part to be willing to change eating habits and lifestyle as part of a treatment program. But attention to these factors can reverse most diseases that plague modern society including arthritis, headaches, multiple sclerosis, hypertension and breast cancer, to name but a few.

As is often the case with physicians who have chosen to explore complementary medicine, my interest in non-mainstream approaches to health care was born from necessity. Within the first several days after the birth of our youngest child, my wife, Leize, began experiencing a variety of problems including severe fatigue, fever, nausea, chills, as well as a peculiar "toxic" body odor. This scenario contrasted vividly with the birth of our first child, when Leize resumed her activities and excellent health almost immediately.

As the problems escalated, we visited her obstetrician who, despite my wife's obvious toxic appearance, tried to assure us that her complaints were of no concern and were typical of the immediate postpartum period. The following day, we met her obstetrician in the emergency room. Even though she was unable to stand, had a high fever, and was unable to tolerate any food or liquid, he decided to place her on an oral antibiotic and, again, sent us home. Two days later Leize sustained a massive hemorrhage, losing two-thirds of her total blood volume. During the short trip to the hospital emergency room, I was truly afraid I would lose her. Upon our arrival, the obstetrician put on a glove and reached into her uterus where he discovered a large piece of placenta that had been mistakenly left behind.

After Leize was finally admitted to the hospital, because of her septic condition, she was placed on very large doses of not one, but three extremely potent antibiotics. Although the rotting fragment of placenta had been removed, her condition continued to deteriorate. Ultimately, she became convinced that she would not survive if she remained in the hospital. After much hesitation, I agreed to honor her wishes and took her home, where I continued to manage her intravenous medications day and night. It soon became clear that she was getting worse with each antibiotic administration. After discussing her case with an infectious disease specialist, the intravenous antibiotics were discontinued and oral medications were begun. But, this did not help either. She was unable to eat and all of her hydration was being provided intravenously.

Finally, one morning she told me, "These drugs are killing me and I don't think I can take much more." She asked me to consult with a homeopathic physician. To say the least, this was very difficult for me to deal with, not only because of my fears of jeopardizing her health but because it flew in the face of all my medical training. Nevertheless, I relented. She began taking a homeopathic thyroid preparation after "muscle testing" by a chiropractor revealed that this would be helpful. Within a few weeks, Leize began to improve, albeit slowly. Soon she was able to walk around the house and tolerate some food. Unfortunately, her condition did not improve further and she remained profoundly weak.

We then began visiting various medical specialists who performed a wide variety of diagnostic tests, all of which revealed that "nothing was wrong." Their ultimate conclusion was that she was suffering from "postpartum depression" and should begin taking antidepressant medications under the direction of a psychiatrist. I had never felt so helpless or isolated. At this point I realized my colleagues could not help us and that we needed to abandon mainstream medicine. We decided to turn things around through our own efforts.

Fortunately, it did not take long to begin finding answers. We soon stumbled upon a fascinating book, *The Yeast Connection*, by William Crook, M.D. It became clear that Leize's main problem was fulminant systemic candidiasis (total body yeast infection), a consequence of the massive doses of antibiotics she had received. I discussed my discovery with several medical colleagues and was very surprised to learn that they considered the idea of "systemic candidiasis" to be foolishness— not a true medical entity. This, in spite of the fact that Leize was demonstrating almost every symptom outlined in a book written by a respected medical doctor! From then on, ignoring the advice of my local colleagues, we started to follow Dr. Crook's program, coupled with the use of homeopathic preparations. Before long, we began seeing a dramatic improvement in her condition.

The road to recovery was long and even after a year, Leize was still not at 100 percent, so we began exploring a wide variety of alternative medical avenues including "live blood cell analysis," a modified Gerson Therapy Program, intravenous vitamins, and spiritual healing with our dear friend, the Rev. Dick Smith. In addition, under the careful guidance of Heather Burch of the Pathfinder's Institute, Leize began utilizing Eidetic Imagery, a very powerful technique developed by Dr. Akhter Ahsen, which provides a deep understanding of the role that past experiences play in influencing an individual's thoughts and actions.

Through trial and error, Leize was able to create a personal program which has successfully returned her to excellent health. She is now feeling well, swimming, running and regularly beating me at tennis.

I am convinced that many of the 25 percent of Americans who regularly utilize "alternative medicine" for health care, do so because of a similar experience in their lives. Incredibly, over 70 percent of these individuals do not discuss their alternative choices with their mainstream physicians. This probably stems from a fear of rejection by their physicians, many of whom categorically reject non-mainstream therapeutic approaches.

What I found most distressing about our ordeal was our physicians' closed-mindedness when we wanted to discuss alternative choices. Most of them chose to recognize only those symptoms of Leize's illness which were within their field of expertise. As the saying goes, "When your only tool is a hammer, every problem looks like a nail." It is so harmful for patients to be told that because their problems do not fit into the well-defined category which that specific physician recognizes, their illness must be psychiatric.

It is my hope that any health care providers who read this book will recognize the need to increase the number of tools in their tool boxes by considering all the healing techniques this world has to offer.

Some of the information in this book comes from research. But overwhelmingly, the most important lessons I have learned have come from my patients, watching what treatments helped them improve. After years of research, one fascinating discovery is that there really is an optimum diet for the human being. The nutritional recommendations for a variety of diseases are remarkably similar. Low fat food, low salt intake, reduction of animal product consumption and certain core vitamins are universally helpful recommendations.

My purpose in creating *LifeGuide* is to give you information that will allow your body to do what it naturally wants -- to be healthy. This first edition of *LifeGuide* explores some of the most common diseases and medical problems experienced by patients. It is by no means complete and future books in this series will explore other areas. In addition to chapters on specific diseases, this edition of *LifeGuide* also examines some of the environmental factors that can be detrimental to good health.

Besides exploring the sources and nature of these hazards, you will find straight-forward common sense information about alternative approaches to nurturing good health rather than waging war on disease.

It is my hope that this information will provide ideas and alternatives which can be shared with open-minded physicians in order to create the optimum plan for your recovery and preservation of good health.

LifeGuide evolved from a weekly health and medical newspaper column that I began writing in January 1992. I thank all of my patients who saved this column and said, "You know, you really ought to write a book."

1

Reclaiming Nature's Message

The Flawed Philosophy of Modern Medicine

These days, books about alternative medical practices are among the most popular titles sold. Some Americans, when hearing the term "alternative medicine" envision techniques or treatment programs which deviate from the norm. These alternative methods are often called unorthodox or nontraditional. However, I feel that modern western "traditional" medicine, with its emphasis on fighting disease rather than fostering health, represents the greatest deviation that the world of healing has ever known.

The premise underlying western medicine is that humans are separate from nature. This flawed philosophy is a relatively recent phenomenon. Until recently, mankind has been perceived as an integral part of the universe. This philosophy persisted in western Europe as late as the Middle Ages. What changed the view of modern man? This change was probably catalyzed by the Protestant Reformation. Having demonstrated his ability to undermine the wide-spread authority of the Roman Catholic Church, western man began to feel that he could take control of the entire physical world. As Beinfield and Korngold stated: "In the Christianity of this new era, the realm of Heaven existed outside of Nature, apart from it, barely within human reach. Earth and Heaven were divided into separate realms. The dark, sinister, mysterious forces of earth were juxtaposed with the enlightened, righteous and supernatural forces of Heaven. Instead of being an ally, Nature became an adversary to be overcome and conquered. Man stood outside of it, apart from and above it. The earth was no longer intimately connected to the life of our own body, instead it became an object that could be manipulated and exploited. Human beings were the battleground in which man and Nature, good and evil, spirit and body, wrestled with each other. A unified reality was sacrificed for dominion over Nature, for technology, for 'progress.'"[1]

So the new mindset of western Europe was one which emphasized the physical nature of the earth and all life upon it. Western man then viewed himself and the world around him as physical, mechanical entities about which he could ultimately obtain complete understanding. René Descartes, a 17th Century French mathematician, is credited with ushering in what we now call the western scientific revolution. Descartes maintained that all nature conformed to mechanical laws and that nature could be viewed as a machine, devoid of both rationality and soul. Unfortunately, this new philosophy became and remains the philosophy of modern western medicine. As Descartes stated, "I do not recognize any difference between the machines made by craftsmen and various bodies that nature alone composes." Or, as Julien Offray de La Mettrie wrote in 1750, "Let us conclude boldly then, that man is a machine."[2]

Understanding the human body and consequently the study of medicine became a very physical pursuit, quite squarely in the domain of the physical scientist. As more and more was learned about the human "machine," God and spirituality became less involved in protection and guidance.

The mechanistic view of the human body was easily validated by the increasingly detailed work of anatomists describing the extremely efficient pump and its associated pipes (heart and circulatory system), the lungs acting like bellows and the nervous system acting like a highly advanced electrical communications network. Western medicine became simply a quest to understand how the human machine functioned. The body was, and continues to be, reduced to structural parts, proceeding from organs to tissues, tissues to cells, cells to molecules, etc..

As elucidated by Sir Isaac Newton, laws governing the activity of the human machine actually governed all physical events. Newton's view of the universe held that there were fixed laws of cause and effect. In the mid 1880's when Louis Pasteur discovered the origin of disease outside the body in the form of germs, the Newtonian law of cause and effect, as it applied to the human machine, was confirmed. Each of the diseases that affected mankind was viewed as having a single external "cause" which led to a specific "effect"—a particular illness. This narrow minded view of disease causation focused only on the external "cause" and failed to consider the total condition of the *person*. Medicine became focused, and even to this day remains focused for the most part, on this single cause idea.

As Larry Dossey, M.D. stated in his inspirational book, *Medicine & Meaning*: "... when humans are seen as machines, it is very difficult for physicians to accept the extraordinary and the unexpected. Machines are deterministic and therefore predictable—one of their essential characteristics is that they 'follow the rules' when they 'get sick,' machines don't experience 'miracles,' 'exceptional cures,' or 'spontaneous remissions.' They don't improve, but only depreciate, break down, wear out and eventually have to be replaced. Their 'clinical course' is always in one direction—toward the junkyard."[3]

Marti Kheel, writing in the *Townsend Letter for Doctors* (January 1992), effectively summarized this viewpoint: "According to this view, nature was a machine, devoid of both rationality and soul. ... The twin notions of conquering nature and viewing nature as machine have become the life-blood of modern western medicine. According to modern scientific viewpoint, disease reflects a failure in the body machine. When disease strikes, it is the body's machinery that must be repaired. Whether the repair takes the form of surgery, drugs, or the replacement of 'defective' body parts, such adjustments must be performed by those thought to have the necessary technology, expertise and skill. ...Animals who were also machines, could experience no pain. Their cries of anguish upon being dissected were mere mechanical responses."[4]

So western medicine has evolved into a system which is essentially based upon fighting a war. We are led to believe that there is a constant assault upon our bodies by a vast array of enemies, constantly seeking an opportunity to disrupt our health. The human body is a battlefield on which western medicine wages its war against disease. Medical students emerge from training understanding the utility of various drugs, which they will use as their weapons in fighting this war. As Kheel points out, two of the weapons used in the war against cancer are nitrogen mustard and radiation, both of which were used as weapons of mass destruction during the last two World Wars.[5] Even the *terminology* of warfare permeates the modern medical arena. We hear of the "war on cancer;" *bombarding* cells with an *arsenal* of drugs, and of *magic bullets* that *target* cancerous tumors. Another phrase we often hear is that a certain medical war will be won—provided, of course, that biomedical research scientists are given sufficient funds.

Even after medical students graduate and begin to practice, they continue to be bombarded by this mentality. Day in and day out, doctors are blanketed by the one illness-one magic drug doctrine. An article in the February 1992 issue of *Consumer Reports* indicates that the pharmaceutical industry spends some $5 billion annually to promote its products to doctors.[6] Doctors are the target of very sophisticated, subtle and highly effective marketing techniques that permeate virtually every aspect of the practice of medicine. Drug companies sponsor all expense paid "symposia" to Caribbean resorts for physicians (and spouses) to learn about new drugs. A recent technique is the "dinner meeting," where drug companies invite physicians to a very expensive restaurant to "discuss" the treatment of a particular disease. Invariably this discussion centers on the use of a specific drug, produced by the dinner host. After the promotional lecture, physicians are given an "honorarium," typically $100, for simply attending.

Until recently makers of the drug Inderal were giving physicians frequent flyer mileage for every Inderal prescription written! Are such marketing techniques effective? Without a doubt. A 1982 study by a Harvard professor, Jerry Avorn, showed that doctors' opinions of two popular, heavily advertised drugs, came directly from the ads and sales pitches. Although the doctors believed their information came from objective scientific sources, those sources, in fact, clearly stated that the drugs were *not* effective for their advertised uses.[7]

Who is subsidizing this highly effective marketing campaign? The American consumer. Between 1980 and 1990, while general inflation was 58%, health care costs rose 117%, and the cost of drugs increased *by an astounding 152%.*[8]

This analysis of the origins and philosophy of modern western medicine will help you see how distinctly it contrasts with "alternative" or "holistic" approaches to health care. To a typical western allopathic physician, a "holistic practitioner" is an oddity—someone way out of the mainstream, practicing unorthodox, "nonscientific," "nontraditional" types of medicine. I am especially intrigued when alternative medicine is called "nontraditional", because this implies that modern western medicine is "traditional." A traditional practice is one that has been accepted or utilized by the majority of a population for a long period of time.

I have often been accused of practicing "nontraditional medicine" because I frequently prescribe herbs and herbal preparations. However, this practice is clearly more traditional. The use of herbs is probably as old as mankind. Historical sites in Iraq show Neanderthal man using yarrow and other healing herbs some 60,000 years ago. In fact, the World Health Organization estimates that even today healing herbs are the primary medicines for 4 billion people, two-thirds of the world's population.[9]

A related discipline which I utilize in my daily practice is Ayurveda. Also considered nontraditional, Ayurveda is derived from the two Sanskrit words: *Ayur*—meaning life, and *veda*—meaning knowledge. Ayurveda (the knowledge of life) has its foundation in the Rig Veda, one on India's classic books of wisdom written some 4,500 years ago. Even to this day Ayurvedic medicine is utilized by some 70% of Indians and Pakistanis. So, it becomes increasingly difficult to classify these alternative approaches to health care as nontraditional.

The holistic philosophy of medicine is based on the premise that the whole person, not simply the symptoms of disease, must be treated. Illness is not conceived as a single disease with a specific cure, but rather as an expression of disharmony with the natural world. The inner environment of the body and outer environment of the surrounding world are seen as one integrated whole. Holistic tradition honors not only the body's power to heal, but that of the mind and spirit as well. Modern holistic medicine has evolved from traditions in which prayers, chants, incantations and other forms of ritual accompanied the preparation and ingestion of herbs and other substances of the earth to augment the body's own healing energy in order to fortify health, rather than combat disease.

In addition to re-establishing harmony in the internal environment (body, mind and spirit), the holistic practitioner recognizes the importance of preserving the external environment. Anthropologist Gregory Bateson summarized our present relationship with our world by stating, "an organism that destroys its environment destroys itself."[11]

Holistic medicine recognizes that a natural environment, uncontaminated food, proper exercise, clean air and clean water are far more influential in fostering health and well-being than prescription drugs. This challenges the very foundation upon which the Western medical industrial complex is based.

Our almost exclusive reliance upon the products of the highly profitable pharmaceutical industry is taking its toll. Kheel reminds us that, "industries continue to pollute our environment with toxic chemicals and drugs while medical scientists continue to refine increasingly potent drugs to 'cure' us of the illnesses that our poisoned environment has produced: pharmaceutical industries bombard both our inner and outer environment with the equally toxic chemicals and drugs."[12] As Hans Rusch stated, "According to the FDA, 1.5 million Americans had to be hospitalized in 1978 as a consequence of taking drugs which were supposed to 'cure' them of something or other. Some 30% of all hospitalized people get further damaged by the therapy that is imposed on them. The number of people killed in the U.S. by the intake of drugs has been estimated at some 140,000 each year."[13]

Our misdirected priorities were well described by Prince Charles when addressing the British Medical Association, saying, "It is frightening how dependent upon drugs we are all becoming and how easy it is for doctors to prescribe them as the universal panacea for all ills. Wonderful as many of them are, it should still be more widely stressed by doctors that the health of human beings is so often determined by their behavior, their food and the nature of their environment."[14]

In keeping with the theme of internal and external harmony, the American Holistic Medical Association defines wellness as "... a state of well-being in which an individual's body, mind, emotions and spirit are in harmony with and guided by an awareness of society, nature and the universe." Wellness medicine "emphasizes personal responsibility and fosters a cooperative relationship among all those involved. ...{it} encompasses all safe modalities of diagnosis and treatment, including the use of medications and surgery, emphasizing the necessity of looking at the whole person, including analysis of physical, nutritional, environmental, emotional, spiritual and lifestyle values."[15]

Preventive medicine is not widely practiced in America for two major reasons. First, preventive medicine is not very dramatic. Giving a patient dietary information which may reduce his or her long-term risk of cardiovascular disease certainly lacks the impact and drama of a coronary artery bypass operation. Yet, despite the fact that coronary artery disease is almost entirely preventable, it still accounts for nearly 40% of total deaths in the United States today. In fact, of the 14 leading causes of death in this country, 11 are directly influenced by lifestyle factors and are highly preventable.[16]

The second, and most important reason preventive medicine lacks popularity is that it's not revenue intensive. For such groups as the pharmaceutical industry, there is little to gain and everything to lose if disease is prevented. The coronary artery bypass operation, which offers recipients no increase in survival rates compared to patients not surgically treated, is a $6 billion a year industry.[17]

The importance of preventive medicine as a cornerstone of a health care system is perhaps best summarized in the *Nei Jing*, a classic Chinese medical text written in the second century BC, which states, "Maintaining order rather than correcting disorder is the ultimate principle of wisdom. To cure disease after it has appeared is like digging a well when one already feels thirsty, or forging weapons after the war has already begun."[20]

Reliance upon highly technical and complicated medical and surgical techniques, with little concern for basic disease prevention, plays a major role in our skyrocketing health care costs. As Robert Anderson remarked, "...since 1970, the cost for medical and surgical management of sick persons in the United States has risen from 7% of the gross national product to 10% at present, costing $355 billion dollars in 1983. One-third of this increased cost was due to the intensity and complicated nature of the services involved."[18] This is an especially telling statement, in light of a recent U.S. government report which stated, "It has been estimated that only 10% to 20% of all procedures currently used in medical practice have been shown to be efficacious by controlled trial."[19]

Whereas modern western medicine is founded upon a distrust of nature and our natural ability to heal, the holistic perspective honors the body's own healing energy, the earth, the mind and the spirit. The entire history of western medicine represents a deliberate and protracted struggle to conquer and subdue the life-giving forces of nature. The holistic approach to health care is becoming increasingly popular as more people seek to reclaim the sense of connectedness with the vital forces of nature. In ancient times our existence was seen as wholly entwined with nature. Earth was looked upon as a true mother, caring for and allowing the symbiotic interaction of all living things.

Within the holistic perspective, humanity cannot be separated from nature. What is beneficial for humanity is beneficial for nature. What destroys nature also destroys humanity. To harm any part of nature is to harm the whole—including humanity. This philosophy is based upon ancient eastern wisdom that all life occurs within the circle of nature and that within this circle all living things are mutually dependent. As Chief Seattle stated in 1854, "This we know—the earth does not belong to man, man belongs to the earth. All things are connected like the blood that unites one family. Whatever befalls the earth, befalls the sons of the earth. Man did not weave the web of life; he is merely a strand of it. Whatever he does to the web he does to himself."[20] In contrast to the modern Western view that mankind exists as an entity apart from nature with nature's role as a subservient source of exploitation, the holistic perspective holds that for health and life to flourish, there must be harmony between mankind and nature. Our goal is to protect human life by preserving and reclaiming the conditions in which life flourishes.

REFERENCES

1.   Beinfield, Harriet; Korngold, Efrem. *Between Heaven and Earth*. (New York, NY. Balentine Books.) p. 18.

2.   Offray de La Mettrie, Julien. *Man: A Machine*. 1750. (G. Smith. London.) p. 50.

3.   Dossey, Larry. *Meaning & Medicine*. (New York, NY. Bantam Books.) p. 122.

4.   Kheel, Marti. *Western Medicine's War Against the Natural World*, Townsend Letter for Doctors. Jan. 1992.

5.   Ibid.

6.   *Pushing drugs to doctors*. Consumer Reports. Feb. 1992. p. 87-94.

7.   Ibid.

8.   Ibid.

9.   Castleman, Michael. *The Healing Herbs*. (Emmaus, Pennsylvania. Rodale Press.) 1991.p. 1.

10.   Op. cit. 1 p. 30.

11.   Op. cit. 1 p. 6.

12.   Op. Cit. 4.

13.   Rusch, Hans. *The Naked Empress*. (Milano, Italy. Civis Publications.) 1982. p. 12.

14.   Fink, John M. *Third Opinion*. (Garden City Park, NY. Avery Publishing Group.) 1988.

15.   American Holistic Medical Association *Guidelines*. (Denver, CO.) May 1978.

16.   Anderson, Robert A. *Wellness Medicine*. (New Canaan, CT. Keats Publishing, Inc.) 1987. p. 2.17. Crampton, Elmer. *Bypassing Bypass*. (Trout Dale, VA. Medex Publishers, Inc.) 1990. p. 23.

18.   Op. cit. 16 p. 5.

19.   Assessing the Efficacy and Safety of Medical Technologies. P.B. 286/929. Office of Technology Assessment. Sept. 1978.

20.   Op. cit. 1 p. 7.

2

Just Say No to Pesticides

Why Organically Grown Foods are Better

As more Americans begin to recognize the dangers of using pesticides in food production, the demand for organically grown produce will increase dramatically.

Organic fruits and vegetables are grown without the use of pesticides. There is no question that the pesticides used on nonorganic produce pose a significant health threat. A recent issue of the California Public Interest Research Group Newsletter reported, "Using data from a 1987 National Academy of Science report on pesticides in our food supply, it has been calculated that the risks posed by cancer-causing pesticides in our food add up to over one million additional cancer cases in the United States population over our lifetimes. Data generated from private laboratory testing in California puts the figures even higher."[1]

The use of pesticides in farming creates at least three major problems. First, many of today's pesticides are "systemic." This means that rather than simply remaining on the outside of the plant, these dangerous chemical compounds actually become a part of the plant and cannot be washed off or removed by peeling. Second, pesticides frequently remain in the environment for a long time. For example, the half life of the popular pesticide *Toxaphene* is fifteen years. This means that fifteen years after Toxaphene is applied, half of the pesticide remains active in the soil.[2] Pesticides accumulate in the soil for years, contaminating lakes and streams, and are frequently found in ground water used for human consumption.

The third major problem is that pesticides may be habit forming to agriculture. As a recent EarthSave Foundation Report reveals, "Unfortunately, due to the remarkable ability of 'pests' to rapidly adapt to toxic chemicals in their environment, more and more pesticides have been needed to produce the same degree of crop protection. Modern agriculture has become addicted to using larger and larger quantities of pesticides that poison the environment and the human food chain."[3] And although pesticide use has increased some 3300% since 1945, crop loss due to insects has actually increased by 20 percent over the same period of time.[4,5] Clearly, we are going in the wrong direction.

The use of pesticides in this country continues to expand.

California farmers alone apply over 400 million pounds of pesticides to their crops every year.[6] But even more alarming is the "circle of poison" created by international pesticide use. Although some of the most dangerous pesticides are now outlawed in the United States, they are nevertheless still produced in the United States and sold to farmers in other countries, primarily Central and South America. As Bill Thomson reported in the January 1991 issue of the *East-West Journal* (now called *East-West Natural Health*), "What these foreign farmers did with the pesticides was their business, reasoned the U.S. manufacturers, who also claimed that the chemicals enabled people to eat who otherwise would not. What the pesticide manufacturers were reluctant to tell American consumers was that many of the foods were grown for U.S. consumption, not to feed the people who grew them. Today, even in the face of this pesticide problem, overall U.S. consumption of fresh fruits and vegetables imported from south of the border has risen to roughly comprise ten percent of our intake, though the figure is even higher in northern regions during the winter."[7]

This completes the circle. We send our highly toxic pesticides abroad where their use is virtually unrestricted. After the produce is harvested, it is exported back to the United States. Much of the produce arriving in the United States goes directly to the consumer without any testing for pesticide residue. On the U.S./Mexican border, for example, only about seven percent of winter fruit and vegetable shipments are checked.[8] And with new trade agreements soon going into effect, the percentage of unchecked produce will likely increase even further.

A shocking amount of America's produce is contaminated by

toxic pesticides. Between 1982 and 1985, a study performed by the FDA found pesticide residues in *48 percent* of the most frequently consumed fruits and vegetables.[9]

Just because a pesticide is manufactured and approved within the United States doesn't necessarily guarantee its safety. As Mary H. O'Brien, information coordinator for the Northwest Coalition for Alternatives to Pesticides, states, "Only 38% of the pesticides on the market in the United States have been tested for cancer-causing ability, as required by law, (i.e., passing two tests). Only 30% to 40% have been tested for birth defects, and less than 10% have been tested for genetic damage."[10]

If the toxicity of nonorganic vegetables is not enough to warrant switching to organically grown produce, consider the fact that organically grown vegetables are generally much higher in various important nutrients. A Rutgers University study comparing organically grown vegetables to typical supermarket produce revealed substantial differences. Organically grown tomatoes, for example, were 500% higher in calcium, 1300% higher in magnesium and an incredibly 193,000% higher in iron, compared to non-organically grown samples. Snapbeans, cabbage, lettuce and spinach were also evaluated with the organic varieties showing similar nutritional advantages.[11]

Fortunately, organic vegetables are appearing in more and more health food stores and in some privately owned supermarkets. Perhaps with enough pressure from consumers, some of the larger chains will be convinced to provide an organic produce section.

Several years ago, before organic vegetables were available in our local stores, my wife organized an organic vegetable co-op.

Several families got together each week and ordered organic vegetables wholesale from a distributor in a nearby city. This allowed us to have organic vegetables at prices almost comparable to supermarket prices. Usually, store-bought organic vegetables cost about twenty percent more than nonorganic selections.

Perhaps the best way to be sure vegetables have not been treated with dangerous pesticides is to grow your own. It really is not that difficult and does not require a lot of space. A small (10 foot x 20 foot) vegetable garden can provide a surprisingly large amount of vegetables. It may not completely supply a family of four, but it certainly can supplement the vegetables obtained from other sources.

In our southwest Florida home, growing vegetables organically is challenging, to say the least. But, through trial and error and a little research, we have been rewarded with a fairly constant supply of nutrient-rich, pesticide-free vegetables, as well as a family project that allows us quality time together.

Of course, we have had problems with insects, but we have learned how to control them, naturally. One of the most fascinating methods we have discovered is introducing "beneficial insects" into our vegetable garden to control pests. There are many kinds of insects that can be used to control a particular pest. Because we grow tomatoes, we ordered *trichogramma*, a tiny wasp that attacks the eggs of moths and butterflies that produce tomato fruit worms and leaf-eating caterpillars. We also introduced lacewing flies whose larvae attack aphids, white flies, mealy bugs, leafhoppers, moth eggs and caterpillars.

Our children were thrilled when the ladybugs arrived. We released 500 ladybugs into the garden and they immediately went to work eating aphids, eggs and larvae of crop-destroying insects. Beneficial insects are easy to purchase by telephone and are very inexpensive. They arrive within two to three days ready to work in your garden. (See resources.)

If you regularly juice fruits and vegetables there are important reasons for choosing organic produce. I frequently recommend a program of organic vegetable juices in the treatment of such problems as migraine headaches, arthritis and even cancer. However, it is important to understand that when you juice vegetables, all of their nutrients, and unfortunately contaminants, are concentrated in the juice. Therefore, I strongly recommend that only organic vegetables be used in any juicing program.

I recently suggested a program of organic vegetable juicing to Bill Pogue, a patient with brain cancer (see Chapter 16). Bill first underwent surgery to remove as much of the tumor as was possible. This was followed by radiation treatment and very potent chemotherapy. After a period of organic vegetable juicing and supplemental vitamins and he wrote: "At first, I thought the juicing concept was silly; however, from my response to the juice, it appears to work quite well in reducing my fatigue and increasing my level of activity. After a few days of taking the juice, I was able to get up quicker and more alert in the morning and go to bed later at night. Prior to the juicing, I was totally wiped out by 6 or 7 p.m. and I am now staying up and watching the late news. It was a struggle to get up and get going in the morning and now I am back after juicing to my original 6 a.m. awakening. I am ready to go and meet the day with a fast pace. The outcome was quite welcome."

LifeGuide

RECOMMENDATIONS

1.   Choose organic vegetables whenever available.
2.   Rinse thoroughly in water: cauliflower, cherries, grapes, strawberries, potatoes, green beans, tomatoes, peppers and eggplant. Discard the outer leaves of cabbage and lettuce.
3.   Peel pears, peaches, apples and cucumbers (if waxed) before consumption. This unfortunately reduces the fiber content of these foods. Wash spinach and broccoli in a mild soap solution, and then rinse thoroughly.
4.   If organic produce is not available in your area, consider organizing an organic vegetable co-op. Find out who supplies a health food store in a nearby metropolitan area, contact the supplier and see if they can arrange a weekly delivery to your co-op.

RESOURCES

Several texts provide important information on the dangers of pesticides in our foods. These include:

1. *Silent Spring* by Rachel Carson. Houghton-Mifflin Publisher, Boston, 1962. Available from Penguin Books, 625 Madison Avenue, New York, NY 10022. Silent Spring was one of the first books written to bring the problem of global pesticide use to our attention.
2. *Thirty-four Pesticides: Is Safe Use Possible?* published by the National Wildlife Federation in 1984, (69T), available from NWF, 1412 NW 16th Street, Washington, DC 20036.
3. *Pills, Pesticides and Profits: The International Trade In Toxic Substances*, edited by Ruth Norris. North River Press, Inc. Publisher, Croton-on-Hudson, New York, 1982, 167 p. Available from Council on International and Public Fairs, 777 United Nations Plaza, New York, NY 10017.
4. *Circle of Poison: Pesticides and People In A Hungry World*, by Wier and Schapiro, Institute for Food and Development Policy, San Francisco, 1981. 99 p. Available from I.F.D.P., 1885 Mission Street, San Francisco, CA 94103.
5. To order beneficial insects for your vegetable garden as well as to obtain information about their use, contact: Rincon Vitova, Tel. 800-248-2847.
6. *Organic Gardening* is a terrific magazine about pesticide-free gardening. It is published nine times a year by Rodale Press, Inc. For a subscription write: Organic Gardening, 33 East Minor Street, Emmaus, PA 18098 or you may phone (215) 967-8154

REFERENCES

1.   California Public Interest Research Group, Facts Sheet: Pesticides in our foods, water and homes. *California Public Interest Research Group Newsletter*. Phone number (212) 278-9244.

2.   O'Brien, M.H. *Why no one can say "Pesticides are safe."* NACP. P.O. Box 375; Eugene, OR 97440.

3.   *Our Food, Our World*. EarthSave Foundation Publisher. Santa Cruz, CA. p. 9.

4.   Pimentel, et. al. *Handbook of Pest Management in Agriculture, 2nd edition*. Boca Raton, FL CRC Press. 1990.

5.   Pimentel, D. Cornell University, as quoted by Lisa Y. Lefferts and Roger Blowbaum. Eating as if the earth mattered. *E Magazine*. Jan-Feb 1992; p. 32.

6.   California Public Interest Research Group, Facts Sheet: Pesticides in our foods, water and homes. = *California Public Interest Research Group Newsletter*. Phone number (212) 278-9244.

7.   Thomson, B. The new organic imports. *East-West Journal*. Jan. 1991; p. 44-68.

8.   Mott, Abraham, M. *Your Daily Dose of Pesticide Residues*. Pesticide Action Network International. Friends of the Earth, San Francisco, CA.

9.   Ibid.

10. O'Brien, M.H. *Why no one can say "Pesticides are safe."* NACP. P.O. Box 375; Eugene, OR 97440.

11. Baer, F.E. Why organic food matters. *The Journal of Sustainable Agriculture*. Feb. 1989; p. 3.

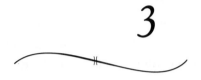

3

The Aluminum Connection

Reducing Your Risk of
Alzheimer's Disease

Alzheimer's disease, or senile dementia of the Alzheimer's type, will be one of America's greatest health problems in coming years. Sixty percent of patients now admitted to nursing homes have this diagnosis, and the number of Alzheimer's victims is projected to increase as much as eight-fold by the middle of the next century.

There is a strong connection between aluminum and Alzheimer's disease. Research clearly demonstrates abnormally high accumulations of aluminum within the brains of Alzheimer's victims. Independent studies performed in Norway, the United Kingdom, France and Canada, show a direct correlation between the prevalence of Alzheimer's disease and aluminum concentrations in the drinking water.[1,2,3,4] In fact, one British study reported in the highly respected medical journal *The Lancet*, showed the risk of developing Alzheimer's disease to be 50 percent greater where drinking water contained high levels of aluminum.[5]

The connection between aluminum in the brain and Alzheimer's Disease is so convincing that various studies are under way to explore whether aluminum in the brain can be removed, and if so, to determine if this would be beneficial for Alzheimer's patients. One fascinating study also reported in *The Lancet*, showed that by administering desferrioxamine, a chemical known to remove aluminum and other metals from the body, the progression of dementia associated with Alzheimer's disease was significantly slowed.[6]

In a recent article appearing in the Townsend Letter for Doctors (November 1993), Dr. Michael A. Weiner, executive director of the Alzheimer's Research Institute, summarized our present understanding of the dangers of aluminum exposure when he stated "... aluminum has been known as a neurotoxic substance for nearly a century. The scientific literature on its toxic effects has now grown to a critical mass. It is not necessary to conclude that aluminum causes Alzheimer's disease to recommend that it be reduced or eliminated as a potential risk. It is the only element noted to accumulate in the tangle-bearing neurons characteristic of the disease and is also found in elevated amounts in four regions of the brain of Alzheimer's patients."

Our exposure to aluminum is certainly nothing new. It is one of the most common elements in the earth's crust and has long made its way into our foods. Ancient man consumed aluminum when rocks were used to mill grain into flour. Minimal exposure to aluminum isn't a problem; our bodies can excrete small amounts very efficiently. Laboratory research has shown that we can handle about twenty milligrams of aluminum ingestion each day.[7] Unfortunately, most of us are exposed to and ingest far more aluminum than our bodies can handle.

What are the sources of aluminum that contribute to toxicity? Aluminum is an ingredient in a wide-range of items that many of us use every day. Some of these products include processed foods, medications and even personal hygiene products.

Aluminum is added as an emulsifying agent in many processed cheeses, especially those which are single-sliced. It is found in cake mixes, self-rising flour, prepared doughs, nondairy creamers, pickles and in some brands of baking powder. Aluminum lauryl sulfate is a common ingredient in many shampoos, while several antidandruff shampoos, including Selsun-Blue, contain magnesium aluminum silicate. Aluminum is an active ingredient in most antiperspirants (aluminum chlorhydrate). However, since people have started becoming more aware of the dangers of aluminum, some "aluminum free" antiperspirants are now being advertised.

Aluminum is readily absorbed by foods cooked in aluminum cookware. In a study conducted at the University of Cincinnati Medical Center, tomatoes cooked in an aluminum pot had a two to four milligram increase in aluminum content per serving.[8]

Perhaps the most significant source of aluminum exposure comes from medications. Most antacid preparations, for example, may contain 200 milligrams or more of elemental aluminum in a single tablet! That's *ten times* more than the presumably acceptable 20 milligrams per day.

This table lists some popular medications containing aluminum:

MEDICATIONS CONTAINING ALUMINUM

ANTACIDS

Di-Gel Liquid	Extra-Strength Maalox Plus
Extra-Strength Maalox	Gaviscon Liquid
Gaviscon Tablets	Gelusil Liquid
Gelusil-II Tablets	Gelusil-II Liquid
Gelusil-M Liquid	Gelusil-M Tablets
Maalox Plus Tablets	Maalox Tablets
Maalox Suspension	Mylanta Tablets
Mylanta Liquid	Mylanta-II Liquid
Riopan	Mylanta-IITablet
Rolaids Antacid Tablets	Tempo Tabs

DIARRHEA MEDICATIONS

Donnagel	Kaopectate
Rheaban	

DOUCHES

Massengill	Summer's Eve

BUFFERED ASPIRIN PRODUCTS

Arthritis Strength Bufferin	Arthritis Pain Formula
Ascriptin	Bufferin
Cope	Vanquish

(From *Drug Facts and Comparisons,* 1991 Edition)

As Dr. Weiner states, "... what is wrong with recommending low aluminum intake as part of an Alzheimer's risk-reduction program? It is a neurotoxic metal of no known use in the human body and is implicated in several other disease states. Before the twentieth century aluminum was not used in any food or pharmaceuticals, and there is no evidence that Alzheimer's disease existed before this century. We are well past the stage of needing to wait for the last double-blinded study before we can recommend preventive steps. There is now enough evidence implicating aluminum in this disease to curtail its intake from all sources."[9]

Although manufacturers of these products may argue that the connection between aluminum ingestion and Alzheimer's disease is not definite, international research proves otherwise. One thing you can do to limit your consumption of aluminum is to *read labels*, especially those of antiperspirants, shampoos, food products and medications. Also reduce your use of aluminum cookware and aluminum foil.

Finally, new scientific research has revealed that it may actually be possible to reduce your absorption of aluminum from dietary and other sources. A study appearing in a recent issue of *The Lancet* reveals that dietary supplementation with a small amount of the trace element silicon (not silicone like in breast implants) can actually, and significantly, reduce gastrointestinal absorption of dietary aluminum.[10]

SOME ANTACIDS THAT DO

NOT CONTAIN ALUMINUM

Advanced Formula Di-Gel Tablets

Alka Seltzer   Alka Seltzer Advanced Formula

Bisodol   Bromo-Seltzer

Rolaids Sodium Free Tablets Titralac Tablets

Tums Extra Strength Liquid

BAKING POWDERS THAT DO

NOT CONTAIN ALUMINUM

Rumford (made from calcium phosphate)

Featherweight   Walnut Acres

Or make your own baking powder from:

2 parts cream of tartar   1 part baking soda

2 parts arrowroot

LifeGuide

RECOMMENDATIONS

1. Avoid all medications, baking powders, and cosmetics that contain aluminum (read labels).
2. Stop cooking in aluminum cookware and using aluminum foil.
3. Drink bottled, distilled, or reverse osmosis processed water.
4. Supplement your diet with silicon (amino acid chelate) 1 mg. each day. Dietary silicon reduces aluminum absorption.

RESOURCES

1. *Prescription for Nutritional Healing.* Garden City Park, New York: (Avery Publishing Group, Inc.). Author James F. Balch, M.D., in his chapter on Alzheimer's Disease, not only describes various sources of aluminum exposure but also presents very useful information about healthful nutritional and herbal supplements.
2. *Beating Alzheimer's* by Tom Warren. This book not only gives important dietary information, but also describes certain chemical allergies that may be important in Alzheimer's Disease.
3. Alzheimer's Disease and Related Disorders Association, 70 East Lake Street, Chicago, IL 60601. (312) 853-3060.
4. Reducing the Risk of Alzheimer's by Michael A Weiner, Ph.D., lists 80 references from mainstream medical literature supporting the link between aluminum exposure and Alzheimer's disease. This book is available by phoning Dr. Weiner at the Alzheimer's Research Institute (415) 388-1006.

REFERENCES

1. Flaten, T.P. An Investigation of the Chemical Composition of Norweigian Drinking Water and Its Possible Relationships With the Epidemiology of Some Disease. Thesis No. 51; Institut of Uorganisk Kjem, Norges Tekniske Hogskole, Trondheim.

2. Alfrey, A.C. "Systemic Toxicity of Aluminum in Man." *Neurobiol Aging* 1986; 7: 543-44.

3. Michel P. Commenges, D. Dartigues and J.F. Gagnon, M, PAQUID Research Group. "Study of the Relationship Between Alzheimer's Disease and Aluminum in Drinking Water." *Neurobiol Aging* 1990; 11: 264 (abstr).

4. Neri, L.C., Hewitt, D. Aluminum, Alzheimer's Disease and Drinking Water. *The Lancet* 1991; 338: 390.

5. Balch, J.F., Balch, P.A. *Prescription for Nutritional Healing.* (Garden City Park, New York. Avery Publishing Group, Inc.)   88-90.

6. Crapper, McLachlan, Dalton, A.J., Kruck, TPA, et al. Intramuscular Desferrioxamine in Patients With Alzheimer's Disease. *The Lancet*, 1991; 337: 1304 1308.

7. Birchall, J.D., Chappel, J.S. Aluminum, Chemical Physiology and Alzheimer's Disease. *The Lancet* 1988; ii: 1008-10.

8. Op. cit. 5.

9. Weiner, Michael A. Evidence points to aluminum's link with Alzheimer's disease. Townsend Letter for Doctors, Nov. 1993, p. 1103.

10. Edwardson, J., Moore, P., Effect of Silicon on Gastrointestinal Absorption of Aluminum, The Lancet, Volume 342, July 24, 1993, pp. 211-12.

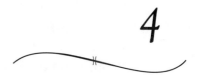

4

Preventing Breast Cancer
The LifeGuide Plan for Improving Your Odds

When I lecture on nutrition and health, I frequently ask audiences what they believe are the best methods for preventing breast cancer. Invariably, one of the answers is: "Women should have frequent mammograms." I am always amused by this response because mammograms have never prevented *even a single case of breast cancer.*

Mammograms are advocated because they can detect breast cancers at an early stage. Actually, by the time a tumor is seen on a mammogram, it has been growing in the breast for about eight years. As medical author Diana Hunt recently reported, "The emphasis that has been placed on mammograms in recent years does a disservice to women. It either lulls them into a feeling of false security—as long as they're having their yearly mammograms, which will detect cancer before it spreads, they think they are safe—or it scares them into thinking that if they don't have a mammogram every year, they will die. The medical profession is boosting 'early detection,' but there is less emphasis on prevention."[1]

I frequently receive literature from groups such as the American Cancer Society (ACS), encouraging me to recommend frequent mammograms for female patients. In fact the ACS recommendations are for women to obtain a baseline mammogram at age 35 years, repeat the examination every year or two between the ages of 40 and 50, and then have a mammogram every year after the age of 50. Most physicians simply reiterate these recommendations to their female patients. As Hunt stated, "...women are encouraged by the medical profession and the X-ray equipment and film manufacturers to have yearly mammograms, in part because of the millions of dollars the procedure brings in every year."[2] Moreover, patients are frequently told that the amount of radiation exposure during a mammogram is minimal. However, mammogram can actually expose women to doses of radiation twenty to twenty-five times greater than an average chest X-ray.[3] This is especially alarming because as John A. McDougall, M.D. has noted, "The human organ most sensitive to the cancer-causing effects of radiation is the female breast. It is even more sensitive than the bone marrow, the lung and the thyroid gland."[4]

The large number of medical clinics specializing in mammography and related services, as well as the "mobile mammography units" often seen at shopping malls, attest to the profitability of this over-utilized procedure. Although mammography can detect tumors earlier than manual breast examination, they fail to detect the presence of a malignancy in twenty-five percent of cases. They also identify as malignant, lumps that are later proven to be benign in up to thirty percent of cases.[5]

Sometimes, it is possible to substitute ultrasound, a technique that does not use radiation, in place of a mammogram. You should certainly ask your physician about this alternative.

In 1992, there were a 186,000 new cases of breast cancer re-ported in the United Stated alone.[7] Despite the technologi-cal advances in mammography and other screening modalities, breast cancer now attacks one woman in nine.[6] The good news is that women *can* dramatically reduce their chances of getting breast cancer. Breast cancer is directly related to fat intake. In countries where women consume lots of animal fat, breast cancer mortality rates are extremely high. For example, in countries like Canada, the United States, Denmark, the United Kingdom and Belgium, where the fat intake is in the 140-180 grams per day range, breast cancer mortality rates are up to 500% greater than in countries like Japan, Costa Rica and Guatemala, where daily fat intake is in the 40-90 gram range.[8] That's why Japanese women have only *one-fifth* as much breast cancer as their American sisters. It's not because they are genetically less susceptible—when Japanese women immi-grate to the United States and adopt our high fat diet, their breast cancer rates skyrocket.[9]

The relationship of dietary fat to breast cancer (as well as cancer of the colon, uterus, cervix and prostate in men) is explained by the following facts. High dietary fat increases the body's production of the sex hormone estrogen, to which breast tissue is remarkably sensitive. It's quite clear that estrogen levels in women are higher now than ever before in the history of mankind. This is demonstrated by the fact that menstruation, brought on by higher levels of estrogen, occurs earlier now than in previous generations. As Neil Barnard, M.D., stated, "According to the World Health Organization, the average age of puberty in girls in western countries in 1840 was about 17 years of age. Today, we take it as a matter of course that girls will reach puberty at 11, 12 or 13."[10] In parts of the world where low fat diets are maintained, the onset of puberty in women still ranges between 15 and 19.[11] The direct relationship between a high fat diet and breast cancer also involves carcinogens (cancer-causing chemicals) in the environment. Since many carcinogens are fat soluble, a diet high in fat encourages absorption of carcinogens and allows them to remain in the body longer, increasing their ability to promote cancer.[12]

Diets high in protein, especially animal protein, are also linked to breast cancer.[13] According to Dr. Barnard, "Research has implicated animal proteins more than other sources of protein. One reason may be the tendency of chemicals such as DDT to concentrate in animal tissues. DDT is still commonly found in meats years after it was banned."[14] DDT, like many other of the so-called "chlorinated pesticides" is one of the most carcinogenic chemicals known to exist. Quite disturbing is recent research revealing that fat from human breast cancer patients has been found to have almost twice of much of some chlorinated pesticides including metabolites of DDT when compared to control populations.[21] A recent study appearing in *Lancet* evaluated diet and breast cancer in Chinese women. It was shown that high intake of animal proteins (especially red meat), was directly related to increased risk of breast cancer, while increased consumption of soya bean proteins significantly lowered the risk.[15] It has been shown that women who eat meat every day have a risk of breast cancer 380% higher than women who eat meat less than once a week! [16]

So the message is simple. To reduce the risk of breast cancer, significantly reduce the amount of fat and animal proteins in your diet. Fortunately, by simply avoiding meat, you can accomplish both. Avoiding meat means not only red meat, but fish and chicken as well. Although poultry and seafood may be lower in fat, they still have high amounts of animal protein which must be avoided. So the best diet for any woman wishing to reduce her risk of breast cancer is a low-fat vegetarian program.

Although the National Cancer Institute recommends a diet with 30 percent fat, a recent Harvard study showed that such a diet does not measurably reduce the risk of cancer.[17] A breast cancer prevention diet should derive only about fifteen to twenty percent of total calories from fat. But keep in mind that even a totally vegetarian diet can still be high in fat. Vegetables oils are essentially pure fat, so frying foods and other uses of vegetable oils in preparing foods can significantly boost the fat content of the diet. How to determine the percentage of dietary calories derived from fat is fully explained in Chapter 17.

I also recommend certain supplements in a breast cancer prevention diet. Vitamins C, E, beta carotene and the trace element selenium are "anti-oxidants." This means that they help the body rid itself of a group of unstable molecules called "free-radicals," which can lead to damage of the DNA and produce malignancy. Indeed, a recent study of some 89,494 women published in The New England Journal of Medicine revealed a significant reduction of the risk of breast cancer in women whose diets were either rich in vitamin A (beta carotene) or who took supplements.[20] I also recommend supplemental zinc and garlic for their immune-boosting properties.

Recently, the FDA approved a large study of the drug Tamoxifen® to determine its effectiveness in the prevention of breast cancer. Some 40,000 women will be placed on this potentially dangerous chemotherapy to determine if it lowers their incidence of breast cancer. Quite frankly, I find this absurd. Since Tamoxifen (trade name Nolvadex) produces uterine cancer in 1.4% of the patients receiving it, there will be about 560 new cases of uterine cancer as a result of this study.[18]

Using a dangerous drug like Tamoxifen to prevent breast cancer typifies the modern western medical approach to disease prevention. If the clinical trials show that there is even a minimal reduction of breast cancer rates in the 40,000 women taking this drug, it will likely receive FDA approval. Shortly thereafter the makers of Tamoxifen will bombard doctors with advertising in medical journals, persuading them to prescribe Tamoxifen to any woman wishing to reduce her risk of breast cancer. This study is supposedly restricted to women who are considered to be "high risk" for breast cancer. Incredibly, as defined by the designers of this study, this includes *any* woman over the age of 60 years. Then, with little persuasion, millions of American women could begin taking a potentially dangerous drug, much to the satisfaction of its manufacturers.

And yet, there are populations of women in this world whose rates of breast cancer are far lower than could ever be achieved by Tamoxifen. Why most women in the world have much less risk of breast cancer than western women is no secret. Their diets are simply lower in fat and animal protein. When dietary improvements can substantially lower the risk of breast cancer, and do so safely, why would anyone choose dangerous drugs?

Each October during National Breast Cancer Awareness Month (NBCAM), women are bombarded with radio, television, newspaper and even promotional videos in an attempt to persuade them that early detection of breast tumors by getting frequent mammograms offers them the best protection against breast cancer. The highly persuasive propaganda put out by the sponsors of BCAM never mentions the well-documented link between DDT (and other dangerous environmental toxins still being manufactured) and breast cancer. Nor is there any mention whatsoever of the importance of dietary modification and vitamin supplementation in reducing breast cancer risk. As one BCAM pamphlet states, "... you can't assume that modifying your diet or lifestyle will make you safe from disease. Early detection is your breast protection."[19]

Are these just glaring oversights, or do the sponsors of Breast Cancer Awareness Month have a hidden agenda? As it turns out, the primary sponsor of Breast Cancer Awareness Month is Imperial Chemical Industries (ICI), one of the world's largest chemical manufacturing companies and a producer of some of the most dangerous environmental toxins known to exist. As medical author Monty Paulsen recently wrote in the Detroit Metro Times (May 19, 1993), "ICI has been the sole financial sponsor of BCAM since the event's inception. Altogether, the company has spent "several million dollars" on the project according to an ICI spokeswoman. In return, ICI has been allowed to approve—or veto—every poster, pamphlet, and advertisement BCAM uses. Not surprisingly, carcinogens are never mentioned in BCAM's widely distributed literature."

To make matters even worse, Zeneca Pharmaceuticals, an ICI spin-off, is the manufacturer of Tamoxifen which, because of its promotion as a preventive drug now is the top-selling anti-cancer drug in the world with annual sales of almost $500 million. As Paulsen states, "... ICI continues to sell almost a half billion dollars worth of treatment each year for a disease that it may be causing by selling billions of dollars worth of toxic chemicals each year. These are the profits of misery." [19]

LifeGuide

RECOMMENDATIONS

1. Eliminate or significantly reduce all animal products.
2. Maintain a low fat diet; 15 to 20 percent of total calories coming from fat.
3. Increase consumption of dietary fiber (grains and legumes).
4. Recommended supplements:
   Beta carotene-25,000 I.U. each day (with food).
   Vitamin E (Carlson brand) 100 IU each day if you are hypertensive—if not, 400 IU each day (with food).
   Vitamin C—(Ester-C) 2,000 milligrams each day.
   Selenium—100-200 micrograms each day.
   Zinc (picolinate)—30 milligrams each day.
5. Avoid caffeine.
6. Do not have a mammogram at any facility in which your radiation exposure will exceed a total of 2 rads.
7. *Do* have a mammogram if you notice a lump, a nipple discharge, inversion of the nipple, skin dimpling or swelling, or unusual prominence of the veins in your breasts.
8. Make sure the facility doing your mammogram is certified by the American College of Radiology. (see resources).
9. Discontinue all alcohol consumption. Having just one drink each day increases your risk of breast cancer by 40 percent, two drinks causes a 70 percent increase, and three drinks a day can actually double breast cancer risks." (Ref. 22)
9. If your doctor recommends a mammogram, ask him or her if an ultrasound (no radiation exposure) might not be useful instead.

RESOURCES

1. Several excellent cookbooks that will introduce you to vegetarianism are: *The Moosewood Cookbook, The Enchanted Broccoli Forrest and New Recipes From Moosewood Restaurant*, all available from Moosewood Cookbook Series: Berkeley, CA. Ten-Speed Press.

2. *McDougall's Medicine: A Challenging Second Opinion* by John A. McDougall, M.D., available from New Win Publishers. 1985. This excellent book very clearly describes the dangers of high fat in the diet and is an excellent resource.

3. To locate a mammographic facility certified by the American College of Radiology call the Cancer Information Service toll free at (800) 4-CANCER.

4. *National Women's Health Network.* This organization was formed 16 years ago by a group of women activists emphasizing women's *health care*—not medical treatment. The goal of this organization is to promote health awareness and prevention—not drugs, surgery and hospitalization. Members receive a bi-monthly newsletter. In addition, this organization publishes several books including the new *Our Bodies, Ourselves Growing Older* and *The Diet Your Doctor Won't Give You.* Their address is National Women's Health Network, 1325 G Street, N.W. (lower level), Washington, D.C. 20077-2052.

REFERENCES

1.   Hunt, D. "Mammogram Alert." *East-West Journal*. Sept-Oct 1991. p. 55.
2.   Ibid.
3.   Ibid.
4.   Ibid.
5.   Ibid.
6.   Barnard, M.D., N.D. "Women and cancer: Opportunities for preven-
      tion." *PCRM UPDATE*. Sept-Oct 1991.
7.   McGuire, W.L., Clark, G.M. Prognostic factors and treatment decisions
      in axillary node negative breast cancer. *N Engl J Med*. 25 June 1992. 3-
      6: No. 6; p. 1756-61.
8.   Wydner, E. Diet and breast cancer in causation and therapy. *Cancer*. Oct.
      1986. p. 1806.
9.   Barnard, M.D., Neil. *Power of Your Plate*. . (Summer-town, TN. Book
      Publishing Co.) 1990. p. 56.
10.   Barnard, M.D., Neil. Women and cancer: Opportunities for prevention.
      PCRM UPDATE. Sept-Oct 1991. p. 2.
11.   Ibid.
12.   Ibid. P. 3.
13.   Armstrong, B., Doll, R. Environmental factors in cancer incidents and
      mortality in different countries, with special reference to dietary
      practices. *Int J Cancer*. 1975. 15: p. 617-31.
14.   Barnard, M.D., Neil. *Power of Your Plate*. Book Publishing Co.
      Summertown, TN. 1990. p. 62.
15.   Lee, H.P., Gourley, L., Duffy, S.W. Dietary effects on breast cancer risk
      in Singapore. *Lancet*. 1991. 337: p. 1197-200.
16.   Hirayama, T. Paper presented at the Conference on Breast Cancer and
      Diet. U.S.-Japan Cooperative Cancer Research Program, Fred
      Hutchinson Center, Seattle, WA. 14-15 March 1977.
17.   Willet, W.C. Dietary fat and risk of breast cancer. *N Engl J Med*. 1987.
      316: p. 22-28.
18.   *Physicians' Desk Reference*. Medical Economics Co., Inc. Oradell, NJ
      07649. 1992. p. 1102.
19.   Paulsen, M., The Politics of Cancer, Utne Reader, Nov/Dec, 1993, pp.
      81-89.
20.   Hunter, D. J., Manson, J. E., et al, A Prospective Study of the Intake of
      Vitamins C, E, and A and the Risk of Breast Cancer, N. Engl. J. Med.,
      Vol. 329, #4, July 22, 1993, pp. 234-40.

REFERENCES

(continued)

21.   Falck, F., Ricci, A., et al, Pesticides and Polychlorinated Biphenyl Residues in Human Breast Lipids and Their Relation to Breast Cancer, Arch ENV Environ Health, 1992; 47:143-46.
22.   Longnecker, M. P., Berlin, J. A., et al, A Meta-Analysis of Alcohol Consumption in Relation to Risk of Breast Cancer. JAMA, 1988, 260:652-6.

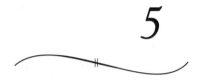

5

Prostatism: A Rite of Passage?
Natural Choices
for a Healthier Prostate

These days, elderly men consider symptoms of prostate gland enlargement to be a rite of passage. This is because so many men in their early sixties suffer from symptoms of prostate disease including frequent interruptions of sleep to urinate, lessening of the force of flow and difficulty starting and stopping urination. These symptoms are a result of gradual enlargement (hypertrophy) of the prostate gland, which causes progressive obstruction of the outflow of urine from the bladder.

The typical approach to prostate enlargement is removing

some or all of the prostate tissue, called prostatectomy. This is a very effective means of relieving most of the symptoms of prostate enlargement, but it's certainly not without risk. According to Dr. Isador Rosenfeld, author of the book, *The Best Treatment*, one-third of all men in the United States have undergone surgical removal of the prostate gland by the time they are eighty-five.[1]   Other techniques designed to reduce the symptoms of prostate enlargement include catheter drainage of the bladder, the use of estrogenic hormones and the use of drugs such as Hytrin and Minipress (both of which reduce blood pressure). These techniques have no effect upon the size of the prostate gland but act only to reduce the symptoms caused by prostate gland enlargement.

There are other ways. For example, many studies have proven that the extract of the berry of a small palm tree known as Serenoa repens (Saw palmetto) to be very effective in treating prostate symptoms. O ne study published in the journal, *Urologia*, evaluated 47 patients with an average age of 65 years who had prostatic enlargement. They received 160 milligrams of Serenoa repens for four months. All of the participants in this study experienced less pain and difficulty with urine flow.[2] Another study conducted in France evaluated 110 patients with prostatic enlargement, one-half of whom received 160 milligrams of Serenoa repens twice a day while the other one-half received a placebo. The group receiving the extract showed significant improvements in symptoms as well as in various measurements of urinary function.[3]

The progressive enlargement of the prostate gland results from accumulations of the male hormone testosterone within the prostate. There, testosterone is converted to a much more potent hormone, dihydrotestosterone (DHT). In the presence of DHT, prostate cells multiply, causing enlargement of the prostate gland. The extract of Serenoa repens prevents the conversion of testosterone to DHT, reducing the amount of this very potent hormone within the prostate gland. Fortunately, the extract of Serenoa repens (Saw palmetto) is now widely available in health food stores. It's a safe, natural and effective way to reduce symptoms of prostate enlargement.

This approach to prostate disease is very effective. I recently evaluated a 63-year-old gentleman who was getting up two to three times every night to urinate. He had no other significant medical problems. He was on no medication, although he did drink two cups of coffee each morning and had an occasional iced tea. He was quite active, biking, walking, and playing golf on an almost daily basis.

His general physical examination revealed nothing remarkable. The prostate examination did show that there was some mild enlargement of the prostate gland on one side but it was soft—a finding indicative of benign enlargement as opposed to malignancy.

I asked him to eliminate caffeine from his regimen, placed him on 2,000 mg. per day of vitamin C, and started him on Saw palmetto.

After two and a half months he was sleeping through the night on most nights or having to urinate just once. He unfortunately did not stop drinking his morning caffeine but did take the vitamin C and Saw palmetto. His response typified the results that we see with the use of this very beneficial herbal supplement.

Essential fatty acids supplementation has been recommended by several medical writers as being helpful for symptoms of prostate enlargement.[4,5]   Like Saw palmetto, essential fatty acid supplements help reduce hormone stimulation of the prostate gland and so reduce prostatic enlargement. This is also the reason a low-fat diet seems to be effective for this problem, since dietary fat increases sex hormone production, stimulating prostate growth.

Supplemental zinc is important for overall prostate health. Zinc deficiency seems to predispose the prostate to infection (prostatitis) which may lead to scarring and prostate enlargement as well.

Various drugs are known to significantly intensify the symptoms of prostate enlargement. These include antidepressants such as Elavil, Sinequan and Tofranil; decongestants like Benadryl and Dimetane; and drugs used in the treatment of Parkinsonism such as Artane and Cogentin. Since these drugs themselves often create difficulties with urination, symptoms may improve if the dosage is reduced or the drugs discontinued.

Finally, keep in mind that cancer of the prostate gland is the third most common malignancy in men. Therefore, if you are experiencing any difficulties with urination, see a urologist immediately for a thorough prostate exam.

LifeGuide

RECOMMENDATIONS

1. Fat reduction. Dietary fat should be reduced to approximately twenty percent of total calories.
2. Try Serenoa repens (Saw palmetto). Take approximately 160 milligrams twice a day. Many preparations of Saw palmetto contain added zinc. If not, add supplemental zinc picolinate, 50 milligrams, to your diet each day.
3. Essential fatty acid supplementation. Take two tablespoons of fresh cold-pressed flaxseed oil each day. This initially may cause some loosening of the stool but typically this problem disappearsafter one to two weeks.
4. Avoid caffeine. This tends to worsen urinary symptoms.
5. Avoid vasectomy. This may lead to various types of prostate problems and *definitely* increases the risk of prostate cancer.
6. Take vitamin B^6–100 mg. each day.
7. Reduce consumption of beer and other alcoholic beverages.
8. Try to keep your serum cholesterol at least below 200 mg/dl.
10. Ask your doctor to check your PSA (prostate specific antigen)—it's a simple blood test. This should be repeated every year or two starting at age 40, and yearly after age 50.
11. Vitamin E (Carlson brand) 100 IU each day if you are hypertensive—if not, 400 IU each day (with food).

REFERENCES

1. Rosenfeld, Isador. *The Best Treatment.* (New York, NY. Book Publishing Co.) 1991.
2. Chirillo-Marucco, E., et al. Extract of Sereona repens (Permixon R) in the early treatment of prostatic hypertrophy. *Urologia.* 5: 1269-77. 1983.
3. Champault, G., et al. Medical treatment of prostatic adenoma. Controlled trial: PA 109 versus placebo in 100 patients. *Ann. Urol.* 18: 407-410. 1984.
4. Walker, M. Serenoa repens extract (Saw palmetto) relief for benign prostatic hypertrophy (BPH). *Townsend Letter for Doctors.* Feb./Mar. 1991. pp. 107-110.
5. Balch, James F., and Balch, Phyllis A. *Prescription for Nutritional Healing.* (Garden City Park, NY. Avery Publishing Group, Inc.) 1990. pp. 271-271.

6

Osteoporosis In Your Future?

Why Calcium Supplements Aren't the Answer

The American public is being bombarded by the media about osteoporosis, and with good reason. Osteoporosis affects some 15 to 20 million Americans,[1] at an estimated cost of $4 billion annually. The United States has the highest rate of hip fractures related to osteoporosis of any developed country in the world.

Why is this so? After all, Americans consume more dairy products than most other people, and we all know that dairy products are an excellent source of calcium, which we are told helps prevent osteoporosis.

Interestingly, there is a direct correlation between the incidence of hip fractures secondary to osteoporosis and consumption of dairy products. Since dairy products are high in protein, our high consumption of these products is one reason the American diet averages about twice as much protein as required. Yet, surprisingly, a diet high in protein, especially animal protein, actually speeds up loss of bone calcium.[2-5] For example, vegetarian women who consume no dairy products or meat have about half the loss of bone calcium by age 65 when compared to nonvegetarian women. "Although biochemists have known for many years that high-protein diets caused bones to lose calcium, this information seems not to get the attention of doctors and patients, most of whom would rather use pills once osteoporosis has developed, than to try to prevent it by modifying patterns of eating and exercise early in life," reports Andrew Weil, M.D.[6]

As protein is broken down into amino acids, it causes the blood to become slightly acidic. To reduce this acidity, calcium is drawn from the bones into the blood stream. This calcium then makes its way to the urine and is excreted. As more protein is ingested, more calcium is lost. John A. McDougall, M.D., states, "Researchers have estimated that doubling the protein in the diet leads to a 50 percent increase in calcium loss in the urine."[7] Not only are animal products (meat, poultry, fish and dairy) dangerous because of their high protein levels, but also because of the kind of protein they deliver. Animal proteins are very high in sulfur compared to vegetable proteins. Sulfur tends to speed up the process by which calcium is removed from the bones and excreted in the urine.

According to the U.S. Department of Agriculture, the trace element boron seems to be highly important in preventing osteoporosis, by slowing down the calcium depletion.[8,9] While meat and dairy products are very poor sources of boron, it is available in a variety of fruits, nuts, vegetables and legumes.

Caffeine consumption has also been shown to significantly increase urinary calcium loss. In fact, drinking several cups of coffee each day may *double* the loss of calcium.[10] Other dietary factors which can speed up the loss of calcium or hinder the amount absorbed include alcohol consumption, excess iron, and diets high in salt or sugar. Certain medications, such as cortisone, various antacids, thyroid supplements and diuretics (water pills) also worsen osteoporosis by speeding loss of bone calcium.

The dairy and nutritional supplement industries have somehow convinced the American population that our epidemic of osteoporosis is related to a deficiency of dietary calcium. We are told to choose one brand of antacid over another because it is "an excellent source of calcium." Even orange juice is now "fortified with calcium." Strange as it may seem, our problems with osteoporosis are not related to any calcium deficiency. We get plenty of calcium—more than enough. As Dr. B. Lawrence Riggs recently reported after completing a study at the Mayo Clinic, "We found no correlation at all between calcium intake and bone loss, not even a trend."[11] And as Weil states, "Osteoporosis is not caused by calcium deficiency in the diet, nor can it be corrected by taking calcium supplements once it develops."[12]

The average American woman consumes 500 to 800 mg of

calcium each day.[13] This far exceeds what the World Health Organization places as the adult minimum requirement at between 400 and 500 mg per day. Experimental research has shown that the daily requirement is actually only 150 to 250 mg per day.[14]

Once it has developed, osteoporosis is very difficult to treat. Recently, the Food and Drug Administration approved the drug Calcitonin, which research has shown to prevent worsening of osteoporosis in approximately 70 percent of patients.

However, the best solution to osteoporosis is prevention, and this requires identifying the cause of the problem. This means, first and foremost, that the diet should be re-evaluated. Animal products such as meat, poultry, fish and dairy products should be significantly reduced if not eliminated. Vegetables high in calcium which include broccoli, soy beans, sunflower seeds, almonds, collard greens, mustard greens, squash, sea vegetables and most legumes, should be favored. Vegetable products such as tofu are also good sources of calcium. Dr. James M. Balch, in his book Prescription for Nutritional Healing, recommends taking up to 3 milligrams of boron daily.[15] Reduce or eliminate consumption of alcohol and caffeine, as well as excess sugar and salt. Finally, a regular program of weight-bearing exercises, including such activities as walking, low-impact aerobics, jogging, dancing and yoga, can definitely reduce bone loss.

LifeGuide

RECOMMENDATIONS

1. Eliminate or significantly reduce all dairy products (milk, cheese, yogurt, butter, cottage cheese, etc.).
2. Reduce or eliminate consumption of animal protein (meat, poultry, fish).
3. Reduce consumption of salt, sugar, coffee and alcohol.
4. Don't take iron unless it is medically necessary. Check your multivitamin to make sure it's iron free.
5. Consume generous quantities of calcium-rich foods including broccoli, soybeans, sunflower seeds, almonds, collard greens, mustard greens, squash, sea vegetables and tofu.
6. Supplement your diet with two to three milligrams of boron each day. Dr. James M. Balch in his book, Prescription for Nutritional Healing, cautions against taking any more than that amount.[15]
7. Engage in a regular program of weight-bearing exercise such as walking, low-impact aerobics, jogging, dancing, or yoga.
8. Take 500-1,000 mg of magnesium (amino acid chelate) each day.

REFERENCES

1.   John Feltman. Prevention's Giant Book of Health Facts.   Rodale Press. Emmaus, PA. 1991.

2.   Kolata, G. How important is dietary calcium in preventing osteoporosis? Science. 1986; 223: p. 519-20.

3.   Zemel, M.B. Role of the sulfur-containing amino acids in protein-induced hypercalciuria in men. J Nutr. 1981; 111: p. 545.

4   Hegsted, M. et. al. Urinary calcium and calcium balance in young men as affected by level of protein and phosphorus intake. J Nutr. 1981; 111: p. 553.

5.   Mazess, R. Bone, mineral content of North Alaskan Eskimos. Am J Clin Nutr. 1974; 27: p. 916-25.

6.   Weil, M.D., Andrew. *Natural Health, Natural Medicine.* (Boston. Haughton Mifflin, Co.) 1990. p. 28.

7.   Barnard, M.D., Neil. *Power of Your Plate.* (Summer-town, TN. Book Publishing Co.) 1990. p.129.

8.   Nielsen, F.H. Boron—an overlooked element of potential nutritional importance. Nutrition Today. Jan-Feb. 1988; p. 4-7.

9.   Nielsen, F.H., Hunt, C.D., et. al. Effect of dietary boron on mineral, estrogen and testosterone metabolism in postmenopausal women. FASEB J. 1987; 1: p. 394-97.

10.   Manahan, M.D. William. *Eat For Health.* (Tiburon, CA. H.J. Cramer, Inc.) 1988. Footnote p. 25, no. 7.

11.   Barnard, M.D., Neil. *Power of Your Plate.* (Summer-town, TN., Book Publishing Co.) 1990. p. 128.

12.   Ibid Reference #6. p. 28.

13.   Manahan, M.D. William. *Eat For Health.* (Tiburon, CA. H.J. Cramer, Inc.) 1988. p. 164.

14.   Nielsen, op. cit. p. 167.

15.   Balch, J.F., Balch, P.A. *Prescription For Nutritional Healing.* (Garden City Park, NY. Avery Publishing Group, Inc.)

7

Milk: Nature's Less Than Perfect Food

How Dairy Products Threaten Health

The American dairy industry has done a magnificent job persuading us that we need all milk and dairy products; that milk is "nature's perfect food." Cow's milk really is a perfect food—but only for baby calves. Among humans, milk and dairy products are responsible for an incredibly large number of health-related problems.

Perhaps the most widely held misconception about milk is its importance for building strong bones in children and helping prevent osteoporosis in the elderly. It does neither. Calcium is certainly very important for proper bone development in babies. But those drinking cow's milk actually absorb less calcium than breast-fed infants, even though cow's milk contains 400 percent more calcium than breast milk.[1] As for osteoporosis in the elderly, hip fractures related to osteoporosis are actually highest in those populations which drink the most milk.[2,4] This is not because milk is low in calcium—it isn't. Unfortunately, the high levels of protein prevent much of this calcium from being absorbed.[3]

As John McDougall, M.D. stated, "The African Bantu woman provides an excellent example of good health. Her diet is free of milk and still provides 250 to 400 milligrams of calcium from plant sources, which is half the amount consumed by western women. Bantu women commonly have ten babies during their life, and breast-feed each of them for about ten months. Even with this huge calcium drain, and relatively low calcium intake, osteoporosis is relatively unknown among these women."[5]

Another reason we are frequently told to drink lots of milk is that it is an important source of vitamin D. Actually, cow's milk is a very poor source of vitamin D. Since the 1930s, vitamin D has been artificially added to milk after it was discovered that vitamin D deficiency was responsible for rickets, a bone development problem among children. There can be problems with vitamin D fortified milk which, by federal regulation, should contain 400 I.U. of vitamin D per quart.[7] One recent report from the *New England Journal of Medicine* described a group of patients suffering from such symptoms as: weakness, decreased memory, constipation, elevated blood calcium, irritability and vomiting. All of the patients were found to have very high levels of vitamin D. This was traced to the milk that they were drinking, which had a vitamin D content of 232,565 I.U. per quart—58,000 *percent higher* than mandated by federal regulations.[9]

Consumption of milk products has been associated with a wide variety of conditions or diseases. In his informative book *Eat For Health*, William Manahan, M.D., indicates that all of the following problems may be related to dairy product consumption: recurring abdominal pain, acne, allergies, anemia, asthma, bed-wetting, behavior problems, blood in stools, colic, colitis, constipation, Crohn's Disease, dandruff, depression, diarrhea, ear infections, fatigue, headaches, hyperactivity, insomnia, joint aches, multiple sclerosis, sinusitis and ulcers. The relationship of milk to most of these problems stems from the presence of milk sugar, lactose, or allergic reactions to some of the proteins found in milk and dairy products.

Many of the gastro-intestinal problems caused by milk consumption are related to the digestion lactose sugar. Most of the world's population cannot tolerate milk products due to a deficiency of lactase, the enzyme required to digest sugar lactose.[10] In many countries, including the Philippines, Japan, Taiwan and Peru, more than 70 percent of the population is lactose intolerant and there is a similarly high rate noted among American blacks.[11] Lactose sugar may even be a problem for people who are not deficient in lactase. A study conducted at Harvard by Dr. Daniel Cramer concluded that lactose may be responsible for the 300 percent higher incidence of ovarian cancer in women who consume dairy products.[12]

Most other health problems caused by dairy products represent allergic reactions to some of the more than sixty types of protein found in milk. Many of these problems are behavioral or involve the nervous system, including migraine headaches, mood disturbances, vertigo, epilepsy, insomnia, nervousness, hyperactivity, poor attention span and excessive periods of sleep.[13]

There is also a strong correlation between milk consumption and the incidence of insulin dependent diabetes.[18] One possible explanation for the higher rates of diabetes among milk drinkers involves milk proteins. These proteins may stimulate the body's own immune system causing destruction of the insulin secreting cells of the pancreas leading to insulin dependent diabetes.[19]

Even the prestigious American Academy of Pediatrics has finally shifted its position cow's milk. It is now recommended that infants under one year of age not receive whole cow's milk at all. This recommendation resulted from studies showing that infants drinking cow's milk run a much higher risk of becoming anemic. As research from the University of Iowa published in the *Journal of Pediatrics* recently revealed, "In a large proportion of infants the feeding of cow's milk causes a substantial increase of hemoglobin loss. Some infants are exquisitely sensitive to cow's milk and can lose large quantities of blood."[27]

Medical literature in the mid-1950s reported that milk drinking is beneficial for patients suffering from a duodenal ulcer.[20] This belief is still widely held despite proof that milk products stimulate greater production of stomach acid, causing duodenal ulcers to heal much more slowly.[21]

So, milk and dairy products are far from being "nature's perfect food," or "too good to be just for the young" as the dairy industry would like us to believe. In my practice, I see problems directly related to milk consumption virtually every day. Children seem to be particularly sensitive to milk and show the greatest positive response when dairy products are removed from their diets completely.

Eliminating dair products often puts an end to frequent ear infections, sinus infections, nasal congestion and upper respiratory tract infections which affect so many people these days, especially children. In addition, children often show dramatic improvements in their ability to concentrate with decreased hyperactivity after dairy products are eliminated.

Finally, perhaps the best reason to avoid dairy consumption is the presence of toxins. Cows eat large quantities of grains treated with toxic chemicals, and their milk often contains significant levels of toxins and contaminates. In addition, dairy cows are frequently treated with high dosages of antibiotics to stimulate growth and to treat infections. Sulfa drugs, tetracyclines and other antibiotics have been found in sixty-three to eighty-six percent of milk samples studied.[22]   As Carol Tucker-Foreman, former assistant Secretary of Agriculture stated, "Two-thirds or three-quarters of all the penicillin and tetracycline manufactured in this country go for some therapeutic use in animal production."[23] So it is important for people who are allergic to antibiotics to realize that they may be present in milk and may lead to severe allergic reactions.[24-26]

LifeGuide

RECOMMENDATIONS

1.   Reduce or eliminate consumption of milk and dairy products.

2.   Increase consumption of calcium-rich foods (See Osteoporosis chapter).

3.   Read labels. Avoid processed foods containing "milk solids" or other dairy derived contents.

4.   Try to get outdoors for a fw minutes each day as sulight allows the skin to produce vitamin D. (This even happens on overcast days and in shady areas.)

5.   Use soy milk or rice milk as substitutes for cow's milk (available at most health food stores).

RESOURCES

1. *Eat For Health*, by William Manahan, M.D., past President of the American Holistic Medical Association, is a wonderful resource. I have been recommending it to my patients for the past several years because the nutritional information is so clearly presented and useful. It can be ordered by contacting: H.J. Kramer, Inc., P.O. Box 1082, Tiburon, CA. 94920

REFERENCES

1. Manahan, M.D., William. *Eat For Health*. (Tiburon, CA. H.J. Cramer, Inc.) 1988; p. 164.
2. McDougall, M.D., John. *cDougall's Medicine: A Challenging Second Opinion*. (Piscataway, NJ. New Century Publishers). 1985; p. 68.
3. Linkswiler, M.M., et. al. Calcium retention of young adult males as affected by level of protein and of calcium intake. Transactions of the New York Academy of Science. 1974; 36: p. 333.
4. Op. cit. Reference 2, p. 68.
5. Mcdougall, M.D., John, McDougall, Mary A. *The McDougall Plan*. (Piscataway, NJ. New Century Publishers). 1983. p. 52.
6. Nielsen, F.H. Boron—an overlooked element of potential nutritional importance. Nutrition Today. Jan-Feb 1988; p. 4-7.
7. Department of Health and Human Services. Grade "A" Pasteurized Milk Ordinance. 21 C.F.R. 131.110. 1989; p. 243.
8. Holic, M.F., Shao, Liuww Q., Chen, T.C. The vitamin D content of fortified milk and infant formula. N Engl J Med. 30 April 1992; 326; No. 18: p. 1178-81.
9. Jacobus, C.H., Holick, M.F., Shao, Liuww Q., et. al. Hypervitaminosis D associated with drinking milk. N Engl J Med. 1992; 326: p. 1173-7.
10. Oski, F.A. Don't Drink Your Milk. Syracuse, NY. Mollica Press. 1983.
11. Ibid. Reference 10, p. 16.
12. Cramer, D.W., et. al. Galactose consumption and metabolism in relation to the risk of ovarian cancer. Lancet. 1989; 2: p. 66-71.
13. Campbell, M.B. Neurologic manifestations of allergic disease. Ann Allerg. Oct 1973; 31: p. 485-98.
14. Balyeat, R.M., Wrinkel, H.J. Allergic Migraine in Children. Amer J Dis Child. 1931; 42: P. 1133-72.
15. Davison, H.M. Allergy of the nervous system. Quart Rev Allerg. 1952; 6: p. 157.
16. Campbell, M.B. Neurologic manifestations of allergic disease. Ann Allerg. Oct 1973; 31: p. 485-98.
17. Monro, J., et. al. Food allergy in migraine. Lancet. 5 July 1980. 2: p. 1-4.
18. Scott, F.W. Cow milk and insulin dependent diabetes: Is there a relationship? Mam J Clin Nutr. 1990; 51: p. 489-91.
19. Barnard, M.D., Neil. *Power of Your Plate*. (Sum-mertown, TN., Book Publishing Co.) 1990. p. 128.

REFERENCES

(Continued)

20. Doll, R., Friendlander, P., Pygott, F. Dietetic treatment of peptic ulcer. Lancet. 1956; I: p. 5-8.

21. Kumar, N., et. al. Effect of milk on patients with duodenal ulcers. Br Med J. 1986; 293: p. 666.

22. Jacobson, Michael, et. al. Safe Food. Venice, CA. Living Planet Press. 1991. p. 77-78.

23. Op. cit. Reference 19. p.106.

24. Vickers, H.R., Bagratuni, L. and Alexander, S. Dermatitis caused by penicillin in milk. Lancet. 15 Feb. 1958. 1: p. 351-52.

25. Zimmerman, M.C. Penicillin: Treatment of 52 patients with allergic reactions to penicillin. Antibiotics Annual. 1957-58. p. 313-320.

26. Wicher, K., Reisman, R.E., Arebesman, C.E. Allergic Reaction to penicillin present in milk. JAMA. 7 April 1969. 208: No. 1. p. 143-45.

27. Ziegler, E.E., Fomon, S.J., Nelson, S.E., et. al. Cow Milk Feeding in Infancy: Further Observations on Blood Loss From the Gastrointestinal Tract. Journal of Pediatrics. 1990; 116: 11-8.

8

Mercury: Toxic Waste in Your Mouth?

The Health Benefits of Mercury-Free Dentistry

Mercury is an extremely powerful biological poison—more toxic than lead, cadmium or arsenic. Yet, more than 85 percent of Americans are constantly exposed to this dangerous element, which makes up about 50 percent of the dental amalgam known as the "silver filling." Each year more than 200 million dental restorations are performed in this country and most of them contain mercury. Unfortunately, only 2 percent of the 150,000 dentists in the United States have recognized the profound danger of mercury and have stopped using it in their dental practices.

Until recently, the American Dental Association maintained that once mercury was combined with other ingredients to form an amalgam filling, it was "locked in" and could not escape. Worldwide studies, however, have demonstrated that a significant amount of mercury vapor does escape from mercury fillings and is absorbed directly into the body. Such activities as chewing, consuming hot or acid foods, or even brushing the teeth causes mercury to be released from amalgam fillings.[1,4] Gargling with a mouthwash containing hydrogen peroxide causes mercury amalgams to become oxidized, greatly increasing the amount of mercury released into the mouth.

According to Dr. Thomas W. Clarkson, writing in the prestigious *New England Journal of Medicine*, "Autopsy data indicate that brain-mercury levels are approximately twice as high in people who have had fillings for many years as in those with no fillings, and those with fillings have elevated blood and urine mercury values as well."[5] We now know that there is a direct correlation between the number of mercury amalgam fillings in the mouth and the amount of mercury found in the brain, kidney and other bodily tissues.[6] Dentists have significantly higher than normal levels of mercury in their pituitary glands[7] and multiple sclerosis patients have eight times higher levels of mercury in their cerebrospinal fluid.[8]

These are not new discoveries. Two thousand years ago the Romans recognized its toxicity when miners were dying of mercury poisoning. Mercury is extremely toxic to the nervous system, causing damage to the nerves and brain.[9] It also causes emotional and behavioral disorders, birth defects, symptoms of multiple sclerosis, as well as dizziness, confusion, psychosis, arthritis, colitis and kidney damage.

In 1991 the Environmental Protection Agency ordered that all mercury be removed from interior latex paint because of the danger of mercury exposure. However, the amount of mercury vapor exposure is greater for a person with amalgam fillings than for one using latex paint containing mercury!

The World Health Organization, when studying the amount of mercury in food (fish), air and water, declared that amalgam fillings are actually the greatest source of mercury exposure for human beings. The International Conference on Biocompatibility of Materials has said, "Based on the known toxic potentials of mercury and its documented release from dental amalgams, usage of mercury containing amalgam increases health risks of patients, and dental personnel."[10]

The EPA has mandated that dental amalgam, once removed from the mouth, must be handled as a "hazardous waste."[11] As Dr. Sandra Denton asks in the Townsend Letter for Doctors, "...What is it about the mouth that makes this same item nontoxic? Or is it possible that the mouths of some 80 percent of Americans with amalgam fillings are in actuality "toxic waste dumps?"[12] It has been estimated that in North America alone some 100,000 kilograms of mercury are used in dentistry each year.[13]

In 1987, the Swedish Health Board declared amalgam "toxic and unsuitable" as a dental filling material. Sweden actually subsidizes the removal of mercury amalgam fillings for its people. Yet, the American Dental Association has stated that any dentist removing mercury amalgam for "health reasons" is guilty of violating its code of ethics.

Fortunately there are various alternative materials available in place of mercury amalgam. These include porcelain, gold, glass and quartz composites. A composite is a filling made up of any of a variety of hard substances like quartz crystal, held together with a plastic resin. When selecting a composite, it is important to make sure that it does not contain other toxins such as barium or aluminum. Composite fillings typically last as long as mercury amalgams—eight and-a-half-years, according to the American Dental Association. Glass fillings may last much longer. Some dentists recommend "biocompatibility testing," before choosing a material for fillings. This is a blood test designed to determine whether a patient is sensitive to a particular material prior to having that material used for fillings. For those who are "environmentally sensitive" this may be a worthwhile procedure, but it costs between $200 and $300.

The removal of mercury amalgam fillings releases a significant amount of mercury into the bloodstream. So it is important to understand how to reduce this risk when the fillings are removed, as well as what to do *before* visiting your dentist to reduce the risk of mercury exposure.

Doctors David J. Ogle and Jonathan V. Wright, at the *Tahoma Clinic* in Kent, Washington, have developed a protocol for patients having mercury fillings removed. Their program involves laboratory examinations of blood, urine and hair; a specific diet; and administration of the "dental amalgam IV." They administer this intravenous solution within two hours before each dental appointment. The solution contains EDTA, a "chelating agent," and vitamin C, which are known to help prevent absorption of mercury during the dental procedure. The intravenous is then repeated immediately following the procedure. As Dr. Donald E. Soley of Reno, Nevada states, "...chelating the patient the day before his amalgams are removed protects him at a time of high exposure. If he has a high level of EDTA in his bloodstream (EDTA remains in the blood around 24 hours), the chelating agent binds to this fresh influx of mercury ions, like handcuffing a criminal."[14]

When mercury fillings are removed, perhaps the most important consideration choosing the right dentist. Ideally, he or she should utilize the following procedures in order to minimize your exposure to mercury. First, because mercury is vaporized as the filling is removed, an oxygen or compressed air mask should be placed over your nose to prevent inhalation. Second, a high volume suction device should be used, also to reduce the possibility of mercury vapor inhalation. Third, it is a desirable to wear protective glasses during the procedure to protect your eyes from small particles of mercury amalgam.

Actions do speak louder than words. I became so convinced about the dangers of mercury amalgam fillings that two years ago I decided to have all of my amalgam fillings removed. I can promise you that this was a strong demonstration of my conviction since sitting in the dentist's chair is perhaps my least favorite activity. Nevertheless, over a period of six months I had all of the mercury fillings removed from my mouth. Before each appointment I self-administered an intravenous chelating solution with vitamin C and magnesium, which was then repeated the day following the dental procedure. After each mercury filling was removed, a glass inlay was bonded in its place.

It is important to remember that there is never a need for dentists to use mercury in your dental care. Discuss the other options outlined in this chapter with your dentist, or locate a dentist who practices mercury-free dentistry (see Resources).

LifeGuide

RESOURCES

1. Environmental Dental Association, toll free: 1-800-388-8123. The EDA offers free information about mercury through dentistry.

2. The International Academy of Oral Medicine and Toxicology, Box 608010, Orlando, Florida, 32860-5831. The IAOMT provides a newsletter to its members as well as a free list of dentists practicing mercury-free dentistry.

3. Queen & Company Health Communications, Inc., Box 49308, Colorado Springs, Colorado, 80949-9308. (719) 598-4968. This company provides a list of mercury-free dentists throughout the United States. The fee is $5.

4. DAMS Newsletter, 725-9 Tramway Lane NE, Albuquerque, NM, 87122. (505) 291-8239. The Dams Newsletter gives information about dentists who practice mercury-free dentistry.

5. *Are Your Dental Fillings Hurting You?* (The Hazards of Having Mercury in Your Mouth!) by Guy S. Sasciana, DMD. This excellent, 300-page book explains the dangers of exposures to dental mercury and is written by a dentist. It is available by sending $14.95 to: Health Challenge Press, Box 39601, Springfield, MA, 01139.

6. To learn more about the mercury toxicity protocol and how to prepare yourself for mercury amalgam removal, call or write Dr Jonathan Wright, Tahoma Clinic, 24030-132nd SE, Kent, Washington, 98042, (206) 631-8920.

RESOURCES

(Continued)

7. It's All In Your Head—Diseases Caused By Silver-Mercury Fillings by Hal A. Huggins, DDS. This wonderful resource book describes a wide range of severe reactions to toxic materials currently used in dentistry. It is available by calling: Huggins Diagnostic Center, 5080 List Drive. Colorado Springs, Colorado, 80919, or call toll free (800) 331-2303.

REFERENCES

1. Svare, C.W. Peterson, L.C. et al. The Effect of Dental Amalgams on Mercury Levels in Expired Air. J. Dental Research. 1981; Vol. 60, No. 9: 1668-1671.

2. Vimy, M.J., Lorscheider, F.L. Serial Measurements of Intra-Oral Air Mercury; Estimation of Daily Dose from Dental Amalgam. J. Dental Research. Aug 1985; Vol. 64 No. 8: 1072-75.

3. Huggins, H.A. It's All In Your Head. 1985. Toxic Element Research Foundation. Colorado Springs, CO.

4. Ziff, S. *Silver Dental Fillings-The Toxic Time Bomb.* (New York, N.Y., Aurora Press) 1984, 1986.

5. Clarkson, T.W. Mercury—An Element of Mystery. New England Journal of Medicine. Oct 18, 1990; Vol. 323, No. 16: 1137-1139.

6. Ogle, D.J., Wright, J.V. Mercury Toxicity Protocol: Preparation and Post-Amalgam Removal Program. Townsend Letter for Doctors. July 1991; 542-543.

7. Nylander, M. Mercury in Pituitary Glands of Dentists. The Lancet. Feb. 22, 1986; 442.

8. Ahlrot-Westerlund. Second Nordic Symp on Trace Elements Human Health & Disease, Odense, Denmark. Nutr Res. Aug. 1987; suppl, 1403.

9. Sharma and Obersteiner. Metals and Neurotoxic Effects; Cytotoxicity of Selected Compounds onChic Ganglia Cultures. J. of Comparative Pathology. 1981; Vol. 91: 235-244.

10. Proceedings of the International Conference on Biocompatibility of Materials, November 1988, in publication currently by Life Sciences Press, Tacoma, WA.

11. Hemenway, Caroline. Amalgam Declared Dangerous. Dentistry Today. Feb. 10, 1989.

12. Denton, Sandra. The Mercury Cover-Up. Townsend Letter for Doctors. July 1990; 4/88-4/92.

13. Hahn, L.J., Kloiber, R., et al. Dental "Silver" Tooth Fillings. Townsend Letter for Doctors. December 1990; 840-841.

14. Heimlich, Jane. *What Your Doctor Won't Tell You.* (New York, NY. Harper Collins Publishers). 1990. p. 129.

9

Cholesterol: The Good, The Bad and The Ugly
Simple Steps to Lower Your Risk of Heart Disease

Lowering cholesterol has become an American obsession. Just walk down the aisle of any supermarket, and you will find countless products advertized as "low in cholesterol." It is well known that elevated blood cholesterol contributes to cardiac disease. In addition to the damage excess cholesterol causes in arteries, it also lead to other problems including gallstones, mental impairment, impotence, kidney disease, high blood pressure, colonic polyps and even cancer.[1-5]

However, despite all of the bad press, cholesterol does play an important role in the functioning of our bodies. Simply stated, cholesterol is necessary for our survival. In addition to aiding the digestive process, it is an essential component of cell membranes and an important precursor of sex hormones. Fortunately, our bodies manufacture all the cholesterol we need. Therefore, except for a very small group of people whose bodies produce too much cholesterol because of an inherited disease, elevated blood cholesterol levels are almost exclusively diet-related.

We frequently hear of "good" and "bad" cholesterol. In slightly more scientific terminology, the "good" cholesterol is known as HDL (high-density lipoprotein). We consider HDL beneficial because it helps prevent the formation of cholesterol plaque in arteries by helping the body eliminate excess cholesterol. On the other hand, LDL (low-density lipoprotein) is the troublemaker in terms of arterial disease, hence the term "bad" cholesterol. Excess LDL stimulates the formation of arterial plaque, closing down the blood supply to various parts of the body. Later in this chapter, we will explore various techniques for both lowering LDL and raising HDL.

A large, landmark study to evaluate the risk of heart attack began in 1949 in Framingham, Massachusetts. Specifically, this ongoing study is correlating the relationship between blood cholesteral levels and the risk of heart attack. Dr. William Castelli, director of the study, states, "We've never had a heart attack in Framingham in 35 years in anyone who had a cholesterol under 150."[6] Achieving a level of 150 may sound impossible to people with cholesterol problems. But it is in the 150 to 160 range that the maximum reduction of cardiovascular risk actually occurs. Unfortunately, the National Cholesterol Education Program indicates that the "safe" level of cholesterol is 200. That's only 11 points below the level for the average American.[7] So even the "average American" needs to lower his or her cholesterol by 40 points to substantially reduce cardiac risk. Simply by lowering cholesterol 1 percent, you will have a 2 percent reduction in heart attack risk.[8]

Obviously, the best way to reduce cholesterol is to stop eating it. Determining which foods have cholesterol is actually quite simple. No plant products (fruits, vegetables, nuts, legumes) have cholesterol. It is found *only* in animal products. Remember that rule. Animal products which are highest in cholesterol include: meat, dairy products, eggs, shellfish and even chicken. Although often recommended as a substitute for red meat because it is lower in fat, chicken does contain about the same amount of cholesterol as beef—25 mg per ounce. Another recommendation we frequently hear is to eat only "lean portions" of meats. According to Neal Barnard, M.D., author of *The Power of Your Plate*, it is these lean portions of meat that are actually highest in cholesterol.[9]

It takes more than just reducing cholesterol consumption to bring your blood cholesterol down to safe levels. The liver manufactures all the cholesterol we require. But saturated fats cause the liver to produce excess cholesterol, leading to elevated blood cholesterol levels. Found in beef, chicken and processed meats such as hot dogs and bologna, saturated fats are often disguised on package labels as "hydrogenated vegetable oils." Although often are advertised as having "no cholesterol," these oils cause the body to increase cholesterol production. This is due to the hydrogenation process. Hydrogenated oils are found in nearly all processed foods including: packaged cereals, baked goods, frozen dinners and snack foods. Even if a label reads, "no cholesterol" in large letters, the fine print may indicate otherwise. Make no mistake, saturated fats and hydrogenated oils directly elevate blood cholesterol levels.

Various drugs can also elevate blood cholesterol levels. These include: steroids such as cortisone and prednisone, oral contraceptives, Sinemet, Lasix and caffeine, which is one of the most widely used drug in America today. In fact, elimination of caffeine from the diet can actually lower blood cholesterol by as much as 13 percent, which lowers cardiac risk by *a healthy 26 percent.*[10,11]

Dietary modification is the key to safe cholesterol reduction. Foods known to lower cholesterol include the type of water soluble dietary fiber found in oatmeal, beans, barley and brown rice. Other foods that may be helpful include: garlic, sea vegetables and foods rich in essential fatty acids like dark green leafy vegetables, seeds and nuts.

There are now a number of so-called cholesterol-lowering drugs on the market. Although these drugs have been intensively advertised by their manufacturers, they should almost never be used. In 1991, a five-year study on the effect of two popular cholesterol-lowering drugs was reported in the *Journal of the American Medical Association.*[13] This carefully conducted study evaluated the effectiveness of two cholesterol-lowering drugs, Atromid-S and Lorelco. Nearly 3,500 business executives were part of the study; some received one drug, some both and a third group received no cholesterol-lowering medication. The

results showed that although use of the drugs did lower cholesterol, the mortality rate from cardiovascular disease was actually 142 percent *higher* in the group receiving these drugs
compared to the group that did not. In addition, there were
13 deaths due to violence (including suicide) in the group receiving these drugs. Cholesterol-lowering drugs are potentially
dangerous and should be used only as a last resort after strin-
gent dietary measures have failed. They have been found to
cause severe liver and other serious life-threatening problems.

In addition to strictly reducing high cholesterol foods and saturated fats, dietary supplementation with niacin can be significantly helpful in cholesterol reduction. Previously, it was
thought that high levels of niacin (from 500 to 4000 mg per
day) were required to have any meaningful impact on cholesterol was thought to be quite high. But a recent issue of the
American Journal of Medicine described several medical problems related to niacin intake at these levels, including diarrhea,
gout, liver disorders, skin flushing, itching, rashes, aggravation
of peptic ulcers and heart rhythm disturbances.[14] Fortunately,
when niacin is combined with the mineral chromium, the
amount of niacin required to lower cholesterol is significantly
less. A combination of 200 micrograms of chromium with only
100 mg of niacin has a significant effect upon cholesterol levels.[15] Chromium and niacin somehow work very well together
to effectively lower cholesterol levels and a chromium and
niacin preparation is now available in most health food stores.

Aside from knowing your total cholesterol level, it is important to understand how you can lower LDL and raise HDL.
In general, factors that elevate *total* cholesterol elevate LDL.

Obesity and tobacco lower HDL, the good cholesterol, while a regular program of aerobic exercise can have the opposite effect. Fortunately, it doesn't take a lot of exercise to meaningfully increase HDL. One good half-hour aerobic workout three to four times each week can greatly help in bringing up HDL levels.

If your total cholesterol level is in the 150 to 160 range, it isn't necessary to pay particular attention to HDL levels. If total cholesterol levels are higher, however, then it's necessary to examine the ratio between total cholesterol and HDL. Having a total cholesterol/HDL ratio of 3.5 or less is adequate. Unfortunately, the ratio for the average American male is 5.1.[16]

Recent evidence suggests that oxidation of LDL which is a byproduct of normal metabolic functions tends to make LDL much more dangerous with respect to atherosclerosis.[18] Recently, two landmark articles appearing in *The New England Journal of Medicine* have demonstrated a profound reduction of risk for coronary artery disease in both males and females taking relatively small amounts of vitamin E.[19,20] Vitamin E is a potent antioxidant. These studies demonstrated that as little as 100 units of vitamin E each day can reduce the risk of major coronary artery disease by as much as 30 to 40 percent. While vitamin E consumption has little effect on cholesterol levels per se, it goes a long way toward accomplishing the same goal—reducing coronary disease risk.

Finally, a meditation program may be helpful in lowering your cholesterol. One Israeli study has demonstrated a significant benefit from the Transcendental Meditation program for patients suffering from high cholesterol levels. Patients in the study group had an average reduction of cholesterol from 255 to 225, while subjects who did not follow this meditation technique showed no significant change.[17]

So, except for a very small number of people with a heredity disease which causes extremely high cholesterol levels, serum cholesterol can be dramatically lowered *naturally* and *safely* — by proper attention to diet, the use of dietary supplements, exercise and meditation.

LifeGuide

RECOMMENDATIONS

1. Significantly reduce or eliminate all animal products (meat, poultry, dairy and fish).
2. Avoid saturated fats (hydrogenated oils). Read labels.
3. Increase water-soluble fiber containing foods (brown rice, grains, etc.).
4. Supplement with:
    Garlic—one or two cloves or Kyolic®—two capsules three times a day.
    Chrome-Mate (chromium and niacin)—one capsule each day.
    Flaxseed oil (a natural source of essential fatty acids)—one tablespoon each day.
5. Do fifteen to twenty minutes of aerobic exercise each day.
6. Learn a meditation technique and practice it regularly.
7. Vitamin E (Carlson brand) 100 IU each day if you are hypertensive—if not, 400 IU each day (with food).

RESOURCES

1. To learn more about vegetarian low-cholesterol cooking, see Resources Section of Breast Cancer chapter, Chapter 4, beginning on Page 33.

2. *With The Grain*, by Helen Hodgson Brown. Carol & Graf Publishers. New York, NY. 1990. This well researched book describes the importance of a grain-based diet not only for problems of high cholesterol but also osteoporosis, cancer and kidney disease.

REFERENCES

1. Balch, J.F., Balch, P.A. *Prescription For Nutritional Healing.* (Garden City Park, NY Avery Publishing Group, Inc.) p. 207.

2. Isles, C.G., Hole, D.J., Gillis, C.R., Hawthorn, V.M., Lever, A.F. Plasma, cholesterol, coronary heart disease & cancer in the Renfrew & Pailsey survey. Br Med J. 1989; 298: p. 920-24.

3. Cowan, L.D., O'Connell, D.L., Criqui, M.H., Barrett-Connor, E., Bush, T.L., Wallace, R.B. Cancer, mortality & lipoprotein levels: The lipid research clinic's program mortality follow-up study. Am J Epidermiol. 1990; 131: p. 468-82.

4. Vatten, L.J., Foss, O.P. Total serum cholesterol & triglycerides & risk of breast cancer: A prospective study of 24,329 Norwegian women. Cancer Res. 1990; 50: p. 2341-46.

5. Buchwald, Henry. Cholesterol inhibition, cancer and chemotherapy. Lancet. 9 May 1992; 339: p. 1154-56.

6. Barnard, M.D., Neil. Power of Your Plate. Book Publishing Co. Summertown, TN. 1990. p. 15.

7. Ibid. p. 17.

8. Lipid Research Clinic's Program. The lipid research clinic's coronary primary prevention trial results, II. JAMA. 2/15; 3: p. 365-74.

9. Op. cit. 6.

10. Forde, A.H., et. al. The Tromso heart study: Coffee consumption and cerium lipid concentrations in men. N Engl J Med. 23 March 1985; 290: p. 893-95.

11. Thelle, D.S., et. al. The Tromso heart study: Does coffee raise your cholesterol? N Engl J Med. 16 June 1983; 308: p. 1454-57.

12. Kinosian, V.P., Eisenberg, J.M. Cutting into cholesterol: Cost effective alternatives for treating hypercholesterolemia. JAMA. 1988; 259: (15); p. 2249-54.

13. Strandberg, T.E., et. al. Long-term mortality after five-year multifactorial primary prevention of cardiovascular disease in middle-aged men. JAMA. 1991; 266: p. 1225-1229.

14. Goldstein, M., Potential problems with the wide-spread use of niacin. Am J Med. 1985; 881: p. 1988.

15. Hackman, R.M. Chromium and cholesterol. Town-send Letter for Doc tors. October 1991; p. 744-48.13.

REFERENCES

(continued)

16. Barnard, M.D., Neil. *Power of Your Plate.* (Summer-town, TN. Book Publishing Co.) 1990. p. 18.

17. Chopra, Deepak. *Perfect Health.* (New York Harmony Books Publisher). 1990. p. 128.

18. Steinberg, D., Parthasarathys, et al, Beyond Cholesterol: Modification of Low-Density Lipoprotein That Increase Its Atherogenicity. N. Engl. J. Med., 1989, Vol. 320, pp. 915-24.

19. Rimm, E., Stampfer, M., et al, Vitamin E Consumption and the Risk of Coronary Heart Disease in Men, N. Engl. J. Med., Vol. 328, May 20, 1993, #20, pp. 1450-56.

20. Stampfer, M., Hennekens, C., et al, Vitamin E Consumption and the Risk of Coronary Disease in Woman, N. Engl. J. Med., Vol 328, #20, May 20, 1993, pp. 1444-49.

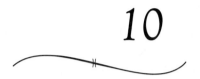

10

Hypertension
Gaining Control of High Blood Pressure

Hypertension, or high blood pressure, is defined as either a systolic pressure (the higher number) over 140, or a diastolic pressure (the lower number) over 90. Hypertension is an extremely common problem affecting some 50 million Americans—20% of our population. Unless high blood pressure is brought under control it represents a major risk factor for such devastating problems as heart disease, stroke, and kidney disease.

Unfortunately, unless the blood pressure is periodically evaluated, there are no warning signs that it may be elevated unless it is very high. At extreme levels of high blood pressure people often experience headaches, nose bleeds, or generalized fatigue. Usually, however, there are no warning symptoms for mild hypertension and that's why it often goes undetected. Mild blood pressure elevation is, nevertheless, very important to recognize as it can lead to progressive damage of the body's arteries, especially those leading to the brain, heart, kidneys, and eyes.

Hypertension may be caused by a variety of medical problems including kidney disease and diseases of the adrenal glands. But, in about 95% of cases, hypertension is essential, meaning that no specific cause can be identified.

Because of the widespread damaging effects of even mild blood pressure elevation, it's important to first recognize the problem, and second, take steps to bring the blood pressure into the normal range. As with so many medical problems, early detection is the name of the game. That means having your blood pressure checked regularly. If you rarely visit a physician, at least take advantage of various other opportunities to have your blood pressure checked. Many drug stores have automated blood pressure testing equipment. Often large shopping malls will offer free blood pressure evaluation on a particular day of the week. I recommend having your blood pressure checked about three or four times each year if it's been in the normal range. Obviously, if your blood pressure is or has been elevated, it should be checked more frequently.

When high blood pressure has been detected, even if mild (diastolic 90-104, systolic 140-149), it should be brought to the attention of a physician. Typically, your doctor should perform the following tests:

> Hematocrit
>
> Urine Analysis
>
> Blood Chemistry Evaluation including:
>
>> Creatinine

Fasting Glucose

Sodium

Potassium

Total Cholesterol

HDL Cholesterol

Red Blood Cell Magnesium Level

Electrocardiogram

These studies are important to determine if there has been any organ damage, to assess overall cardiovascular risk status, and to determine whether or not the hypertension is essential. Your physician may be unfamiliar with a "red blood cell magnesium level." That is because most doctors simply check a serum magnesium level. But, in reality, that makes little sense. Magnesium, one of the most important minerals for energy utilization, is for the most part only found within cells. That's why measuring the red blood cell magnesium level gives a much clearer indication of magnesium status.

The initial approach for lowering mild hypertension should emphasize dietary and lifestyle modification rather than medication, as recommended by the Joint National Committee on Detection, Evaluation, and Treatment of High Blood Pressure.[1] Various studies have shown that a significant weight reduction can be beneficial in reducing the blood pressure. Medical author Larry Katzenstein reviewed five different studies on weight loss and hypertension and stated: "Losing 20 pounds resulted in a decline of 6.3...in systolic and 3.1...in diastolic pressure."[2] He indicated that although these reductions may sound minimal, actually lowering the blood pressure just a few points does significantly reduce the heart attack and stroke risks and may also reduce the amount of medications required. Dr. Norman Kaplan of the University of Texas indicates that half of all hypertensive people are overweight and that there is a direct correlation between weight gain and blood pressure increase.[3] Next, reducing dietary sodium may play a very important role in overall blood pressure reduction. Americans consume lots of sodium, averaging 8 to 10 grams of salt each day. Several large studies have shown significant blood pressure reduction in patients who reduced their sodium consumption to 2 or 3 grams per day.[4,5,6] But it takes more than simply removing the salt shaker from the table. Sodium is found in many foods, especially those which are commercially prepared. Other hidden sources of sodium include monosodium glutamate (MSG), baking soda, and even some medications such as ibuprofen (Advil and Nuprin). Foods high in sodium include diet soft drinks, soy sauce, meat tenderizers, pickled foods, and canned vegetables.

Other dietary recommendations strongly supported by medical literature include: increasing dietary fiber[7,8,9], vegetarianism[10,11,12], and a diet low in fat[13,14]. In addition to a high fiber diet with plenty of fruits and vegetables Dr. James Balch, author of the book, *Prescription for Nutritional Healing,* recommends avoiding aged cheeses, aged meats, and chocolate. He also recommends supplementing the diet with two tablespoons of flaxseed oil each day. That's because flaxseed oil is a very rich source of omega-3 fatty acids. These are the same fatty acids found in the healthful fish oils that we've been hearing a lot about over the past several years. Omega-3 fatty acid supplementation clearly has a beneficial role in an overall plan to reduce high blood pressure[15,16,17].

Other healthful dietary supplements include coenzyme Q_{10}, potassium, and calcium[18].

Lifestyle modification is also an essential component of the hypertensive program. Various meditation techniques have proven their worth in reducing blood pressure. Without question the most widely studied meditation technique is Transcendental Meditation (TM).

In his inspirational book, *Perfect Health,* Dr. Deepak Chopra describes a study at Harvard Medical School in which patients taught the TM technique were found to have an average lowering of blood pressure from 150/94 to 141/88 over a time period ranging from one month to five years[19.] Transcendental Meditation is practiced worldwide and is a very simple technique to learn. In addition to lowering blood pressure, TM has been found to be helpful in lowering cholesterol and reducing various parameters of aging.

Biofeedback is another technique which directly utilizes the "mind-body connection" and like TM and other meditation techniques it has shown its effectiveness in blood pressure reduction[20].

If the blood pressure remains elevated despite these techniques, then it's reasonable to consider a medication. Once a medication has been started it's critical to monitor carefully the blood pressure so that it is not allowed to go too low. A recent study in the *Journal of the American Medical Association* suggested that lowering the diastolic pressure below 85 may actually increase the risk of heart attack. As Kaplan recently indicated in an article in *Annals of Internal Medicine,* "Few physicians are aware that an increasing number of hypertensive patients are being placed at physical risk and made increasingly uncomfortable because of unbridled enthusiasm to "get the pressure down.'" [21]

The most commonly used drugs for controlling blood pressure are: diuretics (water pills), beta blockers, calcium channel blockers, and a group called ACE inhibitors. Interestingly, although the calcium channel blockers such as Cardizem, Procardia, Isoptin, and Calan, as well as the ACE inhibitors such as Capoten, Monopril, Altace, Zestril, and Vasotec lower blood pressure, these drugs may not actually lower the risk of stroke and heart attack. The diuretics and beta blockers, however, not only lower blood pressure, but also achieve the goal of lowering stroke and heart attack risks[22].

Finally, it's important to realize that certain medications prescribed for other medical problems may lead to hypertension. These include antihistamines and oral contraceptives. As Kaplan notes: "As many as 5% of women who take estrogen-containing oral contraceptives and a somewhat smaller percentage of pregnant women, will develop reversible hypertension."[23] One-third of these women will continue having hypertension even after the oral contraceptive is stopped because of damage to blood vessels caused by that hypertension. Hypertension, even if mild, represents a significant health risk. Dietary and lifestyle modifications are sensible first approaches for the mildly hypertensive patient. And if you're already taking a blood pressure medication, these recommendations may allow you to reduce your dosage under the direction of your physician.

LifeGuide

RECOMMENDATIONS

1. Reduce salt consumption to about 2-3 grams per day. Unfortunately, only about half of hypertensives are "salt sensitive" which means that they will have any significant response to salt elimination.

2. Dietary modifications should include increasing fiber (grains and legumes), reducing meat and animal product consumption (total vegetarian diet is best), and reducing total dietary fat.

3. Take fresh cold-pressed flaxseed oil, 1-2 tablespoons per day.

4. Stop cigarette smoking.

5. Discontinue the use of oral contraceptives.

6. Try to reduce your weight to the normal range.

7. Reduce stress and practice a meditation technique such as Transcendental Meditation (TM) or Biofeedback.

8. Garlic (Kyolic®) - 2 capsules twice a day.

9. Coenzyme Q_{10} - 50 milligrams each day.

10. If medication is required, ask your physician to begin with a diuretic (water pill) or a beta blocker. Caution: Beta blockers may elevate cholesterol, and diuretics will likely deplete magnesium and potassium.

11. Calcium - 1,000-1,500 mg per day.

12. Add chelated magnesium 500 to 1,000 mg. to your vitamin program. You may need even more depending on your red blood cell magnesium level.

13. Aerobic exercise (walk, swim, bike, jog).

14. Ester-C (vitamin C) 2,000 mg. per day.

RESOURCES

1. To find a Transcendental Meditation (TM) Center in your area, call (800) 843-8332. I recommend reading Dr. Deepak Chopra's description of Transcendental Meditation in his book, *Perfect Health,* widely available in book stores and also available by calling (800) 255-8332.

2. To find a Biofeedback Therapist, contact: Biofeedback Certification Institute of America, 10200 West 44th Ave., Suite 304, Wheat Ridge, CO., 80033. Telephone (303) 420-2902.

3. The Power of Your Plate, by Neil D. Barnard, M.D., is a terrific "how to" book for those needing information about increasing dietary fiber, lowering dietary fat, and vegetarianism. I order this book 30 copies at a time and distribute it to virtually all of my office patients. It's available by writing Physician's Committee for Responsible Medicine, P.O. Box 6322, Washington, DC, 20015. Or you may call (202) 686-2210.

REFERENCES

1. Katzenstein, L. Your blood pressure - How low can you go? American Health. June 1992. pp. 59-64.

2. ibid, Reference 1.

3. ibid, Reference 1.

4. Kawasaki, T., et al. The effect of high-sodium and low-sodium intakes on blood pressure and other related variables in human subjects with idiopathic hypertension. Am. J. Med. 64: 193-98. 1978.

5. Nonpharmacological approaches to the control of high blood pressure. Final report of the Subcommittee on Nonpharmacological Therapy of the1984 Joint National Committee on Detection, Evaluation, and Treatment of High Blood Pressure. Hypertension. 8 (5): 444-467. 1986.

6. Grobbee, D.E.; Hoffman, A. Does sodium restriction lower the blood pressure? Br. Med. J. 293: 27-9. 1986.

7. Burr, M.L., et al. Dietary fibre, blood pressure, and plasma cholesterol. Nutr. Res. 5: 465-72. 1985.

8. Anderson, J.W. Annals Int. Med. May, 1983.

9. Silman, A.J. Dietary fibre and blood pressure. Br. Med. J. January 26, 1980. pp. 250.

10. Rause, I.L., et al. Vegetarian diet, blood pressure, and cardiovascular risk. Aus. N. Z. J. Med. 14 (4): 439-43. 1984.

11. Rause, I.L, et al. Blood Pressure lowering effects of a vegetarian diet: Controlled trial in normotensive subjects. Lancet. 1: 5-9. 1983.

12. Ophin, O., et al., Am. J. Clin. Nutr. 37: 755-762. 1983.

13. Iacono, J.M., et al. Effect of dietary fat on blood pressure in a rural Finnish population. Am. J. Clin. Nutr. 38 (6): 860-69. 1983.

14. Puska, P., et al. Controlled randomized trial of the effect of dietary fat on blood pressure. Lancet. 1: 1-5. 1983.

15. Norris, P.G., et al. Effective dietary supplementation with fish oil on systolic blood pressure in mild essential hypertension. Br. Med. J. 293: 104. 1986.

16. Singer, P., et al. Lipid and blood pressure lowering effect of mackerel diet in man. Arteriosclerosis. 49 (1): 99-108.1983.

17. Lorenz, R., et al. Platelet thromboxane formation and blood pressure control during supplementation of the Western diet with cod liver oil. Circulation. 67 (3): 504-11. 1983.

18. Werback, M.R. Nutrition Influences on Illness. Keats Publishing, Inc. New Canaan, CT.1988. pp. 227-240.

REFERENCES

(continued)

19. Chopra, Deepak. Perfect Health. Harmony Books. New York, NY. 1990. pp. 127-129.
20. Lock, Steven, and Colligan, Douglas. The Healer Within. Mentor Publishing Company. New York, NY. 1986. pp. 120.
21. ibid. Reference 1.
22. ibid. Reference 1.
23. Kaplan, Norman M. Management of Hypertension. 2nd Edition. Creative Infomatics, Inc. Durant OK, 1987. pp. 19.

11

Why Lose Sleep Over Insomnia?

Natural Choices for a Good Night's Rest

Chronic insomnia, or habitual sleeplessness, is most often a *symptom* rather than a specific disease. According to the American Sleep Disorders Association, more than 35 million Americans report difficulties with sleeping every night, on most nights, or at least several times each month.

The best way to deal with insomnia is to identify and eliminate its cause without resorting to medications. Unfortunately, nonprescription sleep medications are among the most consumed over-the-counter drugs in America today. Products like

Sominex and Nytol can cause a wide range of problems such as confusion, agitation, dryness of the mouth and worsening of urinary difficulties in men with enlarged prostates. Prescription sleep medications are even more dangerous. Halcion, one of the most popular, has been shown to cause confusion and even amnesia. Because of the possible link between severe psychiatric problems and the use of Halcion, its manufacture has been banned in Great Britain. Dalmane, Restoril, Nembutal, Seconal and Valium may also lead to confusion as well as prolonged sedation and drug dependency.

When searching for the causes of insomnia, one of the first places to look is the medicine cabinet. A wide variety of medications contain stimulants which lead to sleeplessness. Among the more common medications that can disrupt sleep are various cold remedies containing decongestants such as pseudoephedrine, appetite suppressants, Dilantin, Inderal and thyroid replacement medications.

Caffeine, even when used only during daytime hours, is one of the most common causes of sleeplessness. Aside from coffee and tea, caffeine is found in chocolate and a wide variety of soft drinks including all cola drinks (except those labeled caffeine free), MR. PIBB, Mountain Dew, Mello-Yello, Tab and Dr. Pepper. Many aspirin preparations and headache remedies also contain large amounts of caffeine. Other caffeine containing drugs include Cafergot, Fiorinal, Soma Compound and Darvon compound.

Often eliminating caffeine consumption is all that is needed to facilitate proper sleep. But that means *total* elimination—no caffeine at all. Many of my patients report problems with insomnia from just one cup of coffee in the morning. That morning caffeine *fix* that so many people are accustomed to, frequently causes what I call the "reverse-rebound effect." The initial stimulating effect of coffee in the morning is followed by a rebound effect of afternoon fatigue that the body then reverses, causing evening stimulation and preventing sleep.

Nervousness brought on by a stressful lifestyle also can make it very difficult to relax and enjoy a good night's sleep. Various stress reduction techniques including progressive muscular relaxation, yoga, T'ai Chi, meditation, deep breathing exercises, biofeedback and guided imagery are all useful in eliminating the buildup of tension. (See Resources in Arthritis Chapter). Ultimately, if insomnia persists despite the utilization of a relaxation technique and caffeine elimination, it might be necessary to change your employment or make some changes in your lifestyle.

Some medical problems, including disorders of the lungs, liver, thyroid gland, muscles and joints, may also disturb sleep by causing pain or discomfort. Eliminating these problems may well eliminate your insomnia.

A crucial consideration is your sleeping environment. Possible causes of sleeplessness include: snoring, excessive movement or sleep talking by your bed partner, an uncomfortable bed, noisy surroundings or even a bedroom that is too quiet.

If your sleeping companion moves excessively in the night a larger bed or separate beds should be considered. Be sure to clearly communicate with your partner about your need for restful sleep. One compromise is having two mattresses side by side on one large box spring. This will allow you to sleep together without having your partner's movements transmitted to your mattress.

Some people are awakened by noises from the street below, the house next door, sirens, etc. But, by the time they are fully awake, they may not remember what caused them to awaken. Conversely, people who have difficulty sleeping in a room that is too quiet may find relief by using a device that creates "background noise" such as a radio playing at low volume, or a machine which creates the sounds of rainfall, a waterfall, or the surf.

When there is no readily identifiable cause for insomnia, various non-medical approaches can be quite helpful . Many studies have shown that the amino acid L-tryptophan is effective in inducing and maintaining sleep. One study reported in the *Journal of the American Geriatric Society*, showed that 30 percent of elderly patients with insomnia had "dramatic and substantial relief" by taking L-tryptophan.[1] Until quite recently, L-tryptophan was widely available and commonly recommended as a sleeping aid. It was recently banned for use in the United States because of some serious health problems possibly stemming from its use. Since L-tryptophan is an amino acid readily found in the human diet, it is unlikely that these reactions were from the L-tryptophan itself. Rather, I agree with Isadore Rosenfeld, M.D., who states, "I suspect it will turn out to have been due to some contaminate in the manufacturing process, and once that's straightened out, L-tryptophan will again be available."[2] Fortunately, certain foods are high in L-tryptophan and thus may help with promoting sleep. These foods include: figs, dates, yogurt, milk and bananas.

On the other hand, foods that should be avoided in the evening hours because they may be stimulating include: cheese, wine, eggplant, potatoes, spinach, alcohol, sugar and caffeine. Although cigarette smoking may seem relaxing, it should be avoided in the evening since nicotine is actually a stimulating drug.

Certain vitamins and minerals may also help induce sleep. Calcium and magnesium work together to allow relaxation of the nerves and muscles. Niacinamide, a form of vitamin B_3, promotes relaxation and may act as a minor tranquilizer.[3] Useful herbs for insomnia include: catnip, skullcap, valerian root and passion flower.

Establishing a routine is often very helpful for the restless sleeper. This includes getting up at about the same time every day, regardless of when you go to bed, getting exercise on a regular basis, and having meals at about the same time every day. Avoid taking a nap during the day.

Exciting new research has revealed the potential usefulness of the hormone melatonin which is contained in the pineal gland of the brain. Melatonin is maximally produced during deep sleep and plays a critical role in mediating the body's normal circadian rhythm as well as in reducing the destructive effect that chronic stress has on the immune system. A small dosage (25 mg.) of melatonin, taken at dinnertime, may prove exceedingly beneficial for the insomniac, especially during stressful periods. Melatonin is at present available only by prescription (see Resources).

Finally, if sleep problems persist, consult a physician who specializes in sleep disorders.

LifeGuide

RECOMMENDATIONS

1. Consider elimination or substitution of any stimulating medication including decongestants containing pseudoephedrine, appetite suppressants, Cafergot, Fiorinal, Soma Compound, Darvon Compound, Vanquish, Midol, Excedrin, Anacin, or any aspirin products containing caffeine. If you take thyroid replacement medication, determine if your dosage is excessive (ask your physician).
2. Eliminate all caffeine consumption, even in the morning.
3. Exercise regularly, preferably during the morning.
4. Avoid daytime naps.
5. Regulate habits: bedtime, wake-up time, exercise, regular bowel movements and meals at approximately the same time every day.
6. Use a relaxation technique such as meditation, guided imagery, progressive muscular relaxation, yoga, T'ai Chi, or biofeedback.
7. Avoid stimulating foods in the evening.
8. Eat foods high in tryptophan in the evening. Such foods include: figs, dates, yogurt and bananas.
9. Try calcium gluconate or calcium lactate (1,000 milligrams) with magnesium gluconate or magnesium citrate (1,000 milligrams) at bedtime.
10. Use helpful herbs, in capsules or tea, including: catnip, skullcap, valerian root and passion flower.

RESOURCES

1. For more information about insomnia contact American Sleep Disorders Association, 1610 NW 14th Street, Suite 300, Rochester, MN 55901. Phone (507) 287-6006.

2. To find a biofeedback practitioner in your area contact: Applied Psychophysiology and Biofeedback, 10200 West 44th Avenue, No. 304, Wheat Ridge, CO 80023. Phone (303) 422-8436.

3. To learn more about herbs in general and how they may assist you with insomnia, I recommend reading the New-Age Herb List: How To Use Herbs For Healing, Nutrition, Body Care and Relaxation by Richard Mabey and Michael McIntyre. New York, NY. Macmillan Publisher. 1988.

4. Your doctor can obtain melatonin by contacting:
   Allergy Research Group
   (510) 639-4572.

REFERENCES

1.   Fitten, L.J., et. al. L-tryptophan as a hypnotic in special patients. J Am
      Geriat Soc. 1985. 33: p. 294.
2.   Rosenfeld, M.D., Isadore. The Best Treatment. (New York, NY. Simon
      & Schuster.) 1992. p. 162.
3.   Mohler, H., et. al. Nicotinamide is a brain constituent with benzodia-
      zephine-like actions. Nature. 1979. 278: p. 563-65.

12

Chelation Therapy
A Safe and Effective Technique for Reversing Heart Disease

In the United States today, more than 40 million men and women are afflicted with coronary artery disease. Each day, heart attacks kill 4,000 Americans—more than 1 million of us each year.

In 1987, more than 330,000 heart patients were subjected to coronary artery bypass surgery in an effort to open up blocked coronary arteries responsible for low blood supply to the heart.[1] Interestingly, various studies have shown that long-term survival and risk of heart attack do not differ when comparing groups of patients treated surgically with those who do not undergo this operation. According to Thomas A. Preston,

M.D., professor of medicine at the University of Washington School of Medicine, "A decade of scientific study has shown that except in certain well-defined situations, bypass surgery does not save lives or even prevent heart attacks. Among patients who suffer from coronary artery disease, those who are treated without surgery enjoy the same survival rates as those who undergo open-heart surgery. Yet, many American physicians continue to prescribe surgery immediately upon the appearance of angina or chest pain."[2]

A nationwide study over ten years at eleven leading U.S. medical centers confirmed that there is no increase in survival rates of patients with coronary artery disease who undergo coronary artery bypass graft (CABG) surgery versus those who do not.[3]

Moreover, coronary artery bypass surgery poses significant physical and emotional risks. As Harvard trained M.D. Elmer Cranton stated in his book *Bypassing Bypass*, "In one to four percent of the cases, depending on the medical center and the surgical team, surgery is fatal, and in up to five percent the surgery itself precipitates a heart attack.   In twenty percent of the cases, serious—sometimes permanent—personality changes result (forgetfulness, irritability, insomnia, inability to concentrate, mental confusion)."[3]

Dr. Cranton's book describes a nonsurgical treatment for coronary artery disease called chelation. This technique involves the administration of an intravenous medicine, EDTA, which is a synthetic amino acid compound. Chelation has been used in the United States in more than 400,000 patients. In 1989, a study by Dr. Efrain Olszewer, published in the *Journal of Advancement in Medicine*, described the results of some 3,000 patients treated with EDTA chelation for coronary artery disease as well as other vascular problems. 90 percent of these patients showed significant improvement.[4]

In describing the usefulness of EDTA chelation, two-time Nobel prize winning scientist Dr. Linus Pauling stated, "Published research and extensive clinical experience showed that EDTA helps to reduce and prevent arteriosclerotic plaques, thus improving blood flow to the heart and other organs. The scientific evidence indicates that a course of EDTA chelation therapy might eliminate the need for bypass surgery. Chelation has an equally valid rationale for use as a preventative treatment."[5]

Even though many scientific studies have confirmed its usefulness of EDTA chelation in improving blood supply to the heart, reducing angina, increasing blood supply to the legs and other vascular problems, it is still not approved by the FDA.[6-8] Why is this so? Simply stated, our profit-driven health care delivery system favors those techniques which produce the greatest revenue. Coronary artery bypass surgery is extremely profitable, not only for the small group of surgeons involved, but also for hospitals and manufacturers of the highly sophisticated equipment used in this procedure. Over $3 billion is spent each year on CABG surgery, although it has not proven to be effective in extending life.

On a positive note, although the FDA has yet to approve EDTA chelation it has approved a comprehensive study of this technique currently under way at Walter Reed Army Medical Center in Washington, D.C., and Letterman Army Medical Center in San Francisco. I'm very confident that the results of this study will be positive and the FDA will be compelled to approve EDTA chelation. Once that happens, private and federal insurance programs will likely provide payment for this highly effective therapy.

In the early 1950s, EDTA chelation was developed as a means of treating patients for toxic metal exposure. Patients exposed to high levels of lead, mercury, or arsenic were given EDTA intravenously because EDTA strongly binds to these toxic metals and allows the body to eliminate them in the urine. It soon became apparent to several doctors using EDTA chelation to treat lead poisoning, that the patients overall health also seemed to improve—especially those with problems related to poor blood supply.[9,10]

After these initial observations were published, several other scientific studies were undertaken that also demonstrated the benefits of chelation therapy. Exactly what followed thereafter is unclear. But it appears that in the early 1960s, the mainstream medical establishment did everything it could to prevent publication of any favorable articles dealing with chelation and discredited it at every opportunity. When supportive studies of the therapeutic benefit of EDTA chelation were submitted for publication in mainstream medical journals, they were uniformly rejected.[11] No doubt the surgical and pharmaceutical industries felt threatened by EDTA and pressured medical journals into suppressing this information. Through their advertising, pharmaceutical companies represent the bulk of revenues generated by medical journals. They often exercise considerable control over what is and what is not published. Since EDTA cannot be patented, there is no great profit to be made; so no pharmaceutical company is interested in marketing it.

How does chelation work? In the presence of certain metals, molecules called "free radicals" are produced within the body. Free radicals are involved in the formation of plaque which occludes blood vessels. It appears that chelation works by removing excess metals from the body, thereby reducing the activity of free radicals and reversing of the process by which artery clogging plaque is produced.

During chelation therapy, patients sit in chairs and receive EDTA (usually with magnesium and vitamin C) intravenously over a period of three to four hours. During the treatment, they sit comfortably, watch television, read, or even sleep. A course of treatments usually involves 20 to 30 infusions and can cost $75 to $120 per infusion. The benefits, however, can be remarkable. Case histories, as reported in Dr. Cranton's book and in Jane Heimlich's, *What Your Doctor Won't Tell You*, attest to the profound effectiveness of chelation therapy. Patients with gangrene, having been told that they must undergo amputation, have chosen chelation instead and have kept their limbs. Patients with crippling angina have become free of chest pain.[12]

EDTA chelation is one of the safest medical therapies ever evaluated. As Dr. Julian Whitaker reports in *Health and Healing*, "...the FDA evaluated the dangers of EDTA chelation therapy. Over the last 30 years, approximately 600,000 patients have had about 12 million EDTA infusions in this country, and the FDA could find no evidence of any significant toxicity. In spite of claims of kidney or other organ damage by opponents of this therapy, the FDA concluded that *safety was not an issue with EDTA*."[13]

In my opinion, chelation therapy is a safe and highly effective treatment option for patients suffering from many forms of vascular disease including: coronary artery disease, angina and poor blood supply to the legs. It also may be useful in the treatment of arthritis, multiple sclerosis, Parkinson's Disease, Alzheimer's Disease, poor healing of wounds and visual problems stemming from inadequate blood supply to the eyes.

RESOURCES

1. *Bypassing Bypass* written by Dr. Elmer Cranton and Arlene Brecher (Donning Co. Publishers. Norfolk, VA) is a must read for anyone suffering from any form of vascular disease and especially for those suffering from coronary artery disease.

2. In *What Your Doctor Won't Tell You* by Jane Heimlich (HarperCollins Publishers. New York, NY) there is a wonderful chapter on chelation therapy that explains fully how chelation was developed and how it is now used. It is an excellent reference book for other problems including hypertension, arthritis and heart disease.

3. To find a qualified chelation practitioner near you, contact: The American College of Advancement in Medicine (ACAM), 23121 Verdugo Dr., Suite 204, Laguna Hills, CA 92653 or call them toll free: 1-800-532-3688 (outside California) or 1-800-435-6199 (in California).

REFERENCES

1. Heimlich, Jane. *What Your Doctor Won't Tell You.* (New York, NY. HarperCollins Publishers). 1990. p. 118.
2. Cranton, Elmer and Arlene Brecher. *Bypassing Bypass.* (Norfolk, VA. Donning Co.) 1989. p. 14.
3. Cranton, Elmer and Arlene Brecher. *Bypassing Bypass.* (Norfolk, VA. Donning Co.) 1989. p. 24.
4. Ibid. p. 11.
5. Cranton, M.D., Elmer. *A Textbook on EDTA Chelation.* (New York, NY. Humay Sciences Press.) 1989. p. 7.
6. Clarke, M.D., Norman E. Treatment of occlusive vascular disease with Disodium Ethylene Diamine Tetra Acetic Acid (EDTA). Am J of Med Science. June 1960. p. 732-44.
7. Casdorph, H.R. Chelation therapy: Efficacy in brain disorders. 1981. 3: p. 101-17.
8. Olszewer, Efrain and Carter, James P. EDTA therapy in chronic degenerative disease. Medical Hypothesis. 1988. 27: p. 41-49.
9. Clarke, Norman E. and Clarke, C. Mosher. Treatment of angina pectoris with Disodium Ethylene Diamine Tetra Acetic Acid. Am J of Med Science. Dec 1956. p. 656-600.
10. Clarke, M.D., Norman E. Treatment of occlusive vascular disease with Disodium Ethylene Diamine Tetra Acetic Acid (EDTA). Am J of Med Science. June 1960. p. 732-44.
11. Heimlich, Jane. *What Your Doctor Won't Tell You.* (New York, NY. HarperCollins Publishers). 1990. p. 123-4.
12. Cranton, Elmer and Arlene Brecher. *Bypassing Bypass.* (Norfolk, VA. Donning Co.) 1989.
13. Whitaker, Julian. Health and healing—Tomorrow's medicine today. Apr. 1992. 2: No. 4. p. 3.

13

Drug-Free
Arthritis Therapy

A Comprehensive
Natural Approach

Arthritis may be the most common disease in the United States today. Characterized by pain and inflammation of the joints, arthritis affects more than 36 million Americans with an annual economic impact of this potentially crippling disease of nearly $14 billion.

Arthritis, which literally means "joint inflammation," actually refers to more than 100 different diseases. However, the two most common varieties are osteoarthritis and rheumatoid arthritis, which afflict 16 million and 2.1 million Americans, respectively.[1] (See Table 1, below).

	OSTEO-ARTHRITIS	RHEUMATOID ARTHRITIS
Age of Onset	Rarely occurs before age 40	Often occurs before age 40
Prevalence in U.S.	16 million	2.1 million
Female:Male Ratio	3:1	2:1 (Juvenile form 6:1)
Joints Involved	Often singular	Typically multiple
Associated Problems	Usually none	Generalized fatigue, anemia, fever and weight loss.
Pain	Mild to occasionally moderate	Often severe and incapacitating
Swelling	Minimal	Often severe

Table 1

Rheumatoid arthritis is by far the more severe of the two diseases. Causing severe pain, swelling and joint deformity, rheumatoid arthritis may also cause total disability. In addition, it is frequently associated with other symptoms including fatigue, anemia, fever and weight loss.

Although osteoarthritis causes minimal pain and disability compared to rheumatoid, it nevertheless represents a significant problem because of the large number of people it affects.

For the most part, medicines used for arthritis are aimed at reducing the symptoms and do nothing to slow the progression of the disease. After trying one arthritis drug after another, without relief, some patients finally begin to explore alternative approaches.

According to the Food and Drug Administration, "Unproven arthritis remedies are among the top ten health frauds in the United States, ... for every dollar that goes to legitimate arthritis research, $25 goes to unproven remedies," states the *Diet & Nutrition Letter*, published by Tufts University.[2]

Nevertheless, I am convinced that many forms of treatment for arthritis, though not part of mainstream medicine, may be extremely beneficial.

An unusual feature of arthritis is that its symptoms vary from day to day. Flare-ups come and go without warning, and sudden improvements may occur without any treatment whatsoever. Therefore, in order to fully assess the usefulness of any new treatment, it must be evaluated over a long period of time—months or even years.

Since all forms of arthritis are characterized by an inflammation, it's useful to examine what inflammation is and how the body controls it. Basically, inflammation is the process by which the body responds to traumas such as injury or infection. Inflammation plays a major role in healing. When an area of the body is traumatized or infected, the inflammation response turns on. Initially, various types of white blood cells migrate to the area. After assessing the situation these white blood cells send chemical signals to all parts of the body causing more specialized white blood cells begin to appear in the injured area. Some types of white blood cells clear away debris such as damaged tissue or infectious bacteria. Others secrete specific chemicals that perform functions such as increasing blood supply, walling off the infection and increasing the temperature in and around the area involved. Once the inflammatory process is fully under way, its five cardinal characteristics—pain, heat, redness, swelling and loss of function—become manifest. These features are present whenever inflammation occurs within the body and are an indication that the body is repairing itself.

Unfortunately, sometimes a full-blown inflammatory response results from very little trauma. This is precisely what happens with arthritis. There is a small degree of trauma associated with the normal wear and tear in joints, but in the arthritic patient, the body over-reacts to these small traumas with an unchecked inflammatory response.

For this reason medical doctors frequently treat arthritis inflammation with steroid anti-inflammatory drugs like cortisone and Prednisone, or nonsteroid anti-inflammatory drugs like Motrin, Naprosyn, Voltaren, Anaprox, Lodine, Orudis, and Relafen. Both groups of anti-inflammatory medications may prove helpful, but not without the risk of serious consequences. Steroid anti-inflammatory medications directly inhibit the immune system and long-term use can cause such problems as cataracts, skin and blood vessel fragility, weight gain, mental changes, atrophy in arms and legs, facial hair growth, worsening of osteoporosis, diabetes and ulcers. Nonsteroid anti-inflammatory medications are not much safer. They can cause a number of problems including stomach ulceration, gastrointestinal bleeding and liver toxicity. Indeed, as the U.S. Food and Drug Administration recently stated, "Two hundred thousand cases of gastrointestinal bleeding, with 10,000 to 20,000 deaths, occur each year due to the 68 million prescriptions of nonsteroidal anti-inflammatory drugs ...used for arthritis."[3]

Obviously, the body must have its *own* ways of reducing inflammation. In fact, the entire process of turning inflammation on and off is controlled by a group of hormones called *prostaglandins*, so named because they were first isolated from prostate gland tissue. How the prostaglandins interact to tightly control the inflammatory response is exceedingly intricate and complicated. Basically, there are two groups of prostaglandins: one group starts inflammation (stimulatory prostaglandins), and one group reduces the inflammatory process (inhibitory prostaglandins).

Through dietary change, the body can stimulate to produce increased levels of inhibitory prostaglandins and, in a very natural way, reduce the excessive inflammation.

All prostaglandins are derived from the fats we eat. The "bad" prostaglandins (stimulatory), which worsen inflammation, are caused by a high fat diet and especially by processed polyunsaturated fats or fats that have been hydrogenated. Since fats exposed to heat become especially troublesome for the arthritis sufferer, frying foods in oil (even vegetable oil) should specifically be avoided. Some fat in the diet is essential, but only the specific type of fat called the *essential fatty acids*. Consuming foods high in essential fatty acids produces more of the inhibitory prostaglandins, thus helping the body reduce inflammation naturally. Foods rich in essential fatty acids include: flaxseed oil (linseed oil), dark green leafy vegetables, black currant oil and evening primrose oil.

Other factors known to enhance the production of stimulatory prostaglandins, which may worsen arthritis, include: alcohol, stress, elevation of serum cholesterol and deficiencies of vitamins B^3, B^6, C or zinc.

Some arthritis sufferers are uniquely sensitive to a group of vegetables called *nightshades*. Nightshades which include green peppers, white potatoes, eggplant, tomatoes and tobacco, contain a toxin called solanine, which in some arthritis sufferers causes increased inflammation and pain.

Norman Childers, M.D., in his book, *Arthritis: Childers' Diet to Stop It*, describes a program which has actually cured some of his arthritis patients and given others much needed pain relief and increased range of motion. This program centers upon eliminating the nightshades. In one study of more than 5,000 arthritic patients over a seven year period, more than seventy percent reported gradual relief from arthritic pain by following Childers' recommendations.[4] Again, keep in mind that it may take several months to determine the effectiveness of such a program.

There are at least three good reasons why arthritis sufferers should eliminate dairy products. First, they are generally high in fat, which, for reasons I've just described, plays a key role in aggravating inflammation. Second, dairy products, especially milk, are often fortified with vitamin D; and vitamin D very specifically intensifies joint pain.[5] Finally, dairy products are the most common cause of food allergies.[6] Various studies have shown food allergies to be directly responsible for worsening of joint pain in arthritic patients.[7,8,9]

Aside from dairy products, other foods known to cause allergic reactions and worsening of arthritis symptoms include coffee, sugar and soy beans. Arthritics also may be sensitive to environmental contaminants including mold, pollen, grasses and certain airborne chemicals.[10] Unless you are suffering from iron deficiency anemia, taking supplemental iron may worsen joint inflammation.[11] Avoid *all* iron supplements completely, even multivitamin supplements containing iron.

Supplemental pyridoxin (vitamin B^6), helps the body produce the inflammation reducing prostaglandins which is helpful for many of the problems associated with arthritis, including pain and stiffness.[12,13] I generally recommend 100 mg of vitamin B^6 twice a day. There is no reason to take more than this amount, and higher dosages may lead to nerve damage.

Other supplements beneficial in the treatment of arthritis include: beta carotene, vitamin E and fairly high dosages of vitamin C. These vitamins are anti-oxidants, which means that they help reduce the joint destruction that accompanies arthritic inflammation.

Two herbs I frequently recommend for arthritis are feverfew and garlic. Both have natural anti-inflammatory effects. Feverfew, in particular, often provides significant pain relief, without the risk of dangerous side effects. This herb should not be taken if you are or may be pregnant.

These dietary measures are often profoundly effective. I recently treated a 63-year-old gentleman suffering from advanced arthritis who had been on prednisone for 18 months. Although he gained some benefit from this medication, it had produced the typical side effects including fungal infections of his fingers and toes. After adopting the dietary program described in this chapter he began showing dramatic improvement. Recently, he wrote, "My arthritis is much better...It is gone from my arms, chest, neck and I have about seventy-five percent relief in my legs. I am now swimming thirty laps in a twenty-five-yard pool each day, whereas, I could only swim four laps, and then was exhausted, before beginning the diet. All muscle fatigue and joint pain have disappeared. The nail fungus on my fingers has been completely cured. The nail fungus on my toes is about fifty percent better. I have gotten rid of all jock itch and ringworm. When I first saw you, I was tired, weak and fatigued. All gone. In fact, my golf game has improved considerably. I am much more alert than I had been and can keep up with the young thirty-five-year olds in the company."

Many of my arthritic patients have also reported good results from acupuncture treatment. A number of patients have reported success with homeopathic preparations. Although I have not been trained in homeopathy, several of my physician colleagues use these preparations quite successfully with their arthritic patients. Since acupuncture and homeopathic medications are safe and have no harmful side effects, they are worth trying.

Regular exercise plays an important role in any arthritis program. Because joint trauma may lead to worsening of symptoms, low- or no-impact activities should be pursued. Swimming is by far the best. Even if you're not a good swimmer, just being in the water is helpful since this eliminates the effect of gravity and allows the joints to relax.

Yoga is also excellent for arthritis sufferers because it is a no impact activity, emphasizing stretching, increasing range of motion and relaxation. Another helpful exercise is T'ai Chi, a very popular Chinese form of movement that was originally a form of self defense. T'ai Chi has evolved into a fitness program using slow, graceful, almost dance-like movements. Like yoga, T'ai Chi is much more than a physical activity. Along with promoting flexibility, coordination and balance, they are wonderful methods of stress reduction, relaxation and meditation. In addition to mobilizing the joints and increasing strength and flexibility, their physical activities help reduce pain by stimulating the production of *endorphins*, the body's natural pain killing chemicals.

Since stress dramatically worsens arthritis, it is essential to adopt a stress reduction program. In addition to T'ai Chi and yoga, one very helpful technique is Transcendental Meditation (TM). More than a million Americans have already been trained in TM, including 6,000 medical doctors. This type of meditation is called "Transcendental" because the mind learns to transcend or go beyond the "noise" of thought to become silent and peaceful. This very simple technique is easily learned and is typically practiced for fifteen to twenty minutes twice a day.

Creative visualization can also be very helpful. One way to use this technique is to hold a specific body part or system in the mind and visualize the healing process. This has lead to decreased pain and swelling for a number of my arthritis patients.

Biofeedback has been used with great success in treating arthritis. This approach reinforces the body's natural mechanisms to help decrease pain and swelling in an affected area.

Those who suffer pain and disability because of arthritis should not give up hope. There are many treatments available without resorting to potentially dangerous drugs. It is likely that one or more of the *LifeGuide* recommendations will prove helpful in relieving your pain, as well as decreasing your reliance upon prescription drugs.

One recent guest on my *LifeGuide* television program was a well-know rheumatologist (arthritis specialist). Throughout the program he maintained that the only treatment for virtually all types of arthritis was the use of pharmaceutical preparations. He adamantly refused to consider that *any* dietary adjustments could affect the course of arthritis. During the program, a member of our studio audience described her long experience with prescription drugs which she had used to treat her arthritis without any benefit whatsoever. Soon after supplementing her diet with vitamin B^6 and zinc, she experienced her first relief in almost 15 years, and has remained symptom-free for two years. Predictably, the rheumatologist maintained that the connection between her recovery and the use of these supplements was "mere coincidence." He felt that because she was no longer taking prescription medications she was missing out on "valuable treatment."

This mentality typifies the narrow-minded approach which so pervades Western medicine today. To enhance the health and well being of our patients, we, as health-care providers, should welcome each other's useful ideas and expand the variety of tools in our toolboxes.

LifeGuide
Recommendations

1. Reduce dietary fat to 15-20 percent of total calories.
2. Decrease or eliminate all processed polyunsaturated fats and hydrogenated fats (read labels).
3. Do not fry foods in oil, not even vegetable oil.
4. Take one tablespoon of flaxseed oil with 500 mg of black currant oil (or 3 capsules of evening primrose oil) twice each day.
5. Try eliminating the nightshade vegetables (white potatoes, eggplant, tomatoes and peppers). Remember tobacco is also a nightshade.
6. Eliminate milk and dairy products.
7. Don't take any supplemental iron unless medically necessary.
8. Do take vitamin B_3, 100 mg daily.
   Vitamin B_6, 100 mg twice per day
   Vitamin C (Ester C with bioflavonoids) 4,000 to 6,000 mg daily
   Vitamin E (Carlson brand) 100 IU each day if you are hypertensive—if not, 400 IU each day (with food).
   Beta carotene, 25,000 units daily (with food).
9. Zinc picolinate, 30 mg each day.
10. Try Garlic, 1 to 2 cloves each day or Kyolic, 2 capsules twice each day.
11. Take Feverfew (made from freeze-dried leaves) 1 capsule two or three times each day. Don't take feverfew if you're pregnant.
12. Adopt a low or no impact exercise program.
13. Try stress reduction meditation (TM), creative visualization, or biofeedback.
14. Consider acupuncture and homeopathic medications.

RESOURCES

1. To learn more about creative visualization contact: Academy for Guided Imagery, P.O. Box 2070, Mill Valley, CA. 94942; area code 415 (393-9324).

2. To find a Transcendental Meditation Center in your area call, toll free (800) 843-8332. A very informative description of Transcendental Meditation can be found in the book, *Perfect Health*, by Dr. Deepak Chopra. (New York: Harmony Books 1990).

3. The book, *Arthritis: Childers' Diet To Stop It*, by Norman F. Childres, Ph.D., describes the Childres program of dietary modification including eliminating the nightshade vegetables. To order, call (904) 372-5077.

4. Basic information about arthritis is available from The Arthritis Foundation, P.O. Box 19000, Atlanta, GA, 30326. Or call toll free (800) 283-7800.

5. To find a biofeedback therapist contact, Biofeedback Certification Institute of America, 10200 West 44th Avenue, Suite 304, Wheat Ridge, CO, 80033. (303) 420-2902.

6. Dr. Mendel's *Lifetime Arthritis Relief System*. (New York, NY: Coward-McCann. 1983). This wonderful book describes simple ways in which foods and chemicals that trigger arthritis pain can be identified and eliminated, and it also describes useful dietary techniques for the arthritic patient.

REFERENCES

1. Balch, J.F., Balch, P.A. *Prescription for Nutritional Healing.* (Garden City Park, NY Avery Publishing Group, Inc.) p. 96.
2. Diet and Nutrition Newsletter. Feb. 1992. 9: No. 12. p. 1-2.
3. Food and Drug Administration press release. Dec. 27, 1988.
4. Childers, M.D., N.F. A relationship of arthritis to the solanacea (nightshades). J Int Cad Prev Med. Nov 1982. p. 31-7.
5. Balch, J.F., Balch, P.A. *Prescription for Nutritional Healing.* (Garden City Park, NY Avery Publishing Group, Inc.) p. 27.
6. Barnard, M.D., Neil. *Power of Your Plate.* (Summer-town, TN. Book Publishing Co.) 1990. p. 132.
7. Brostoff, J., Scadding, G.K. Complexes in food-induced arthralgia. Paper presented at the XII International Congress of Allergy and Clinical Immunology, Washington, DC. Oct 1985.
8. Denman, A.M., et. al. Joint complaints and food allergy disorders. Ann Allergy. 1983. 51: p. 260-3.
9. Mandell, M., Conte, A.A. The role of allergy in arthritis, rheumatism and polysymptomatic cerebral, visceral and somatic disorders: A double-blind study. J Int Acad Prev Med. July 1982. p. 5-16.
10. Heimlich, Jane. *What Your Doctor Won't Tell You.* (New York, NY. HarperCollins Publishers.) 1990. p. 139.
11. Balch, J.F., Balch, P.A. *Prescription for Nutritional Healing.* (Garden City Park, NY Avery Publishing Group, Inc.) p. 98.
12. Ellis, J.M. Vitamin B6 deficiency and rheumatism. Anabolism. Winter 1985.
13. Weil, M.D., Andrew. *Natural Health, Natural Medicine.* (Boston. Haughton Mifflin, Co.) 1990. p. 315.

14

What's Causing Your Headache?

How to Identify and Eliminate Migraine Triggers

Forty-five million Americans suffer from chronic headaches. Although there are various types of headaches, ninety percent are classified as *tension* headaches, caused by tensing the muscles of the back of the neck or head. Typically, the pain of a tension headache is felt in the back of the head or neck, although it may involve both sides of the head, especially in the region of the temples.

The other important headache category is the *vascular* headache, caused by the closing and subsequent opening of the blood vessels in the neck and head. Vascular headaches afflict fewer people, but the pain and disability they cause is often very severe. Commonly described as throbbing, the pain is often one-sided, and frequently accompanied by nausea and vomiting. *Migraine* headaches fall into this category.

According to a recent study in the *Journal of the American Medical Association*, some 8.7 million American females and 2.6 million males suffer from migraine headache. Women between thirty to forty-nine years of age were most likely to require emergency care for acute migraine headaches.[1] Interestingly, about eighty-five percent of women who report migraine headaches had mothers who also suffered from migraines.

These headaches may be preceded by transient neurologic problems such as visual disturbances, numbness or weakness of an arm or leg, difficulty speaking, confusion, smelling strange odors, and even hallucinations. Such symptoms or prodromes normally precede migraine headaches by ten to sixty minutes.

One of the first questions I am asked by headache patients is whether they will need to undergo a brain scan (CAT scan or MRI scan). Typically this question arises from fear that a brain tumor or other serious problem is responsible for the headaches. Unfortunately, it has become almost standard practice for physicians to order a brain scan (which may cost more than $1,200). Often such tests are not necessary if an appropriate history is taken and complete physical and neurological examinations are performed.

Certainly headaches may be indicative of a brain tumor or

other serious problem, but there are several clues which should alert a physician that further investigation is required. These include headaches: (1) that are progressively worsening; (2) that awaken the patient at night; (3) that increase in frequency; (4) that have changed location; (5) that appear for the first time after the age of 40; (6) that appear in patients suffering from other medical problems (such as malignancies or serious infections); (7) that are accompanied by (not preceded by) neurologic problems such as weakness or numbness of an arm or leg, change in vision, difficulty in concentrating, etc.

A brain scan is completely justified when a physical examination demonstrates evidence of improper functioning of the nervous system (weakness, numbness, confusion, visual change, etc.) or increased pressure in the head (determined by eye examination).

Once it has been determined that a headache is not the result of a brain tumor or similarly severe problem, numerous options are available to discover the possible cause and to begin treatment.

The best approach to the treatment of headaches is prevention, and this requires identifying the cause of the problem. Tension headaches are most commonly caused by stress. Some fortunate individuals seem to be able to handle overwhelming stress without consequence. Others internalize even minor stress, and manifest it by tightening the muscles of the head and neck. One technique for reducing muscular tension is regular exercise. The best exercises for tension reduction are aerobic and low-impact; those exercises that cause strain, such as weight lifting or push-ups, should be avoided. As medical writer Nell Hampton recently stated in *Vegetarian Times*, "Another way is to go out and play. I don't mean exercise—I mean play. Fly a kite or build snow people with your kids. Play charades or cards. Having fun is the ultimate stress reducer."[2]

Other useful techniques for stress reduction include: regular meditation, biofeedback, T'ai Chi, hypnotherapy and progressive muscular relaxation.

Some tension headaches result from stress-induced *bruxism* (clenching of the jaw). Unfortunately, many individuals clench their teeth during sleep and don't know it. They often awaken in the morning with a severe headache of both temples with no apparent cause. Simply becoming aware of this often leads to improvement as patients learn to consciously avoid clenching. This problem may also be alleviated by wearing a custom-made bite guard during sleep. An examination by a dentist or oral surgeon may reveal a particular wear pattern of the teeth, suggesting nighttime bruxism, or the diagnosis may be suggested by an observant sleeping companion.

Fortunately, migraine headaches are often brought on by various *triggers* which can usually be identified through persistent investigation. Avoiding these triggers can often lead to a meaningful reduction of migraine frequency. Certain foods which contain high levels of the amino acid *tyramine* are known to trigger migraine headaches. These foods include: chocolate, aged cheese, alcohol (especially red wine), yogurt, liver, vinegar, citrus fruits and yeast extracts. Another very common culprit is caffeine, perhaps the most widely used drug in America today. In addition to coffee, high levels of caffeine are found in chocolate, tea and soft drinks, as well as some over-the-counter pain medications.

Several years ago, while treating a three-year-old boy who suffered from frequent severe headaches, I asked his mother about any possible sources of caffeine. We discovered that he was drinking two cans of cola each day. This may not seem like much of a problem until you realize that the amount of caffeine this thirty-five-pound child was ingesting each day was equivalent to an adult drinking sixteen cups of coffee! In addition to the headaches, he slept poorly, frequently wet the bed, was irritable and had a very poor appetite. Within four days after caffeine elimination, his headaches disappeared, he slept through the night and became a much more pleasant child.

It is very important to read soft drink labels. In addition to cola drinks, you will discover that Mountain Dew, sugar-free Mr. PIBB, Mello-Yello and TAB are among the worst offenders when it comes to caffeine. If you suspect caffeine may be triggering your headaches, try eliminating it completely from your diet.

People who regularly consume caffeine may experience a "rebound headache" or worsening of their headache problem one to three days after caffeine is eliminated. In addition, they may feel weak, irritable, or nauseous for a few days after this toxin is eliminated. During the first week after caffeine cessation, it is important to drink lots of water, take 100 milligrams of vitamin B^6 and 6,000 milligrams of vitamin C each day. This should help reduce the discomfort from caffeine withdrawal.

In a recent article in the journal, *Headache*, Richard Lipton, M.D., showed that Aspartame (NutraSweet) may be a dietary trigger of migraine headaches. In his study of 171 headache patients, 8% reported headaches precipitated by Aspartame.[3] In fact, the Food and Drug Administration has received hundreds of complaints Aspartame causes headaches as well as other neurologic symptoms. According to William Manahan, M.D., author of the book, *Eat For Health*, other problems that may be related to Aspartame consumption include: seizures, depression, memory loss, mood swings, itching, nausea and skin rashes.[4] Unfortunately, Aspartame is now found in a wide array of products including various "sugar-free" foods, wine coolers, laxatives, multivitamins, yogurt and nonprescription drugs.

Another widely used food additive known to trigger migraine headaches is monosodium glutamate (MSG), found in a wide variety of food, including Chinese restaurant dishes. Examples include: frozen dinners, potato chips, various salad dressings, mayonnaise and incredibly, even some baby foods. Also watch out for ingredients such as hydrolyzed vegetable protein, "natural flavor," hydrolyzed plant protein, autolyzed yeast and sodium caseinate—these may contain MSG and are frequent additives to various food products.

Beginning in May 1993, food product labels must comply with new FDA regulations requiring disclosure of MSG and MSG-containing ingredients. Be on the alert for labels that say "contains glutamate."

Many migraine headaches result from sensitivity to certain foods. In one study reported in the journal, *Annals of Allergy*, eighty percent of the patients achieved "major improvement" when foods to which they were sensitive were eliminated from their diets.[5] Food sensitivity often plays a crucial role in children suffering from migraine headaches.[6] Foods which may negatively impact migraine sufferers include: milk products, wheat, chocolate, eggs and bananas. Try eliminating all of these from your diet for three weeks. Then, re-introduce them one at a time to determine which may be causing headaches.

Other common migraine triggers include: cigarette smoking, exposure to second-hand smoke, excessive hunger, lack of sleep, too much sleep, exposure to strong perfumes and emotional stress. Some people are sensitive to sulfites (a chemical used to keep restaurant salads looking fresh) or nitrates (preservatives used in hot dogs and luncheon meats). Certain medications known to trigger migraine headaches include birth control pills, estrogen replacement therapy and, ironically, some headache preparations that contain caffeine.

While certain foods may cause migraine headaches, others may help reduce headache frequency and severity. At the top of this list are foods which contain high levels of omega-3 fatty acids (dark green leafy vegetables, garlic, lima beans, figs and apricots, as well as deep-water fatty fish). In studies performed at the University of Cincinnati College of Medicine and the State University of New York, patients receiving omega-3 fatty acid supplements had significant reductions in frequency and severity of migraine headaches, compared to patients receiving a placebo.[7,8] Fresh cold-pressed flaxseed oil is the best natural source of omega-3 fatty acids.

"Susan" is an active 49-year-old woman I recently treated for intractable headaches. Although she had suffered from headaches *every day* since the age of 19, for over a year they had been growing increasingly more intense. She had undergone CAT scans, MRI scans, an extensive battery of blood work, and many other "tests" at a number of major medical institutions. Doctors had prescribed all kinds of drugs including Inderal, Elavil, Depakote, Cafergot, and Lithium, to no avail. At one point she did use several herbs but they produced only minimal benefit. She had tried an "elimination diet" as well as acupuncture, biofeedback, and even temporal mandibular joint manipulation, but all these treatments proved fruitless. Her medical history revealed that she had suffered from no significant illnesses in the past, although at times she did have peculiar swelling of her hands and feet. Although she neither smoked cigarettes nor consumed alcohol she did consume minimal amounts of caffeine. She exercised quite frequently, enjoying bike riding on an almost daily basis.

Nothing remarkable was noted on her examination although she seemed quite tender to the touch all across the scalp. I placed her on a program including supplemental Vitamin C, E and B Complex, together with beta carotene, magnesium, flaxseed oil and evening primrose oil, and asked her to keep a diary of her headaches.

At a follow up appointment five weeks later, she indicated that for the first time in 30 years she was absolutely headache-free. She began feeling significantly better within three weeks after starting the program and by the fourth week her headaches were completely gone. She remains headache-free.

The combination of flaxseed and evening primrose oil exerts a powerful anti-inflammatory effect by reducing the inflammation of blood vessels in the scalp. Magnesium supplementation is beneficial as well, working with the oils to reduce inflammation. I suspect that she was magnesium deficient because of the history of frequent swelling of the ankles and wrists. Like her headaches, that problem has not returned.

Another dietary supplement which has received considerable recent attention is feverfew, a small, daisy-like flower used in migraine treatment and prevention for centuries. I have found this herb to be extremely helpful for many of my patients. In a recent study reviewed in the *British Medical Journal,* feverfew was found to reduce migraine frequency by more than half.[9] In another study, 70% of the 270 patients reported significant relief, whereas standard medical treatment had provided little or no relief.[10] This herb is now widely available in capsule form. Feverfew has a long folk history as a menstruation promoter, so it should probably not be taken by pregnant women. Also, people taking anticoagulant medications or have a blood-clotting disorder, should consult a physician before using this herb. Other useful herbs for migraine patients include ginko biloba extract, peppermint and rosemary.

Several of my patients have experienced significant relief from chronic headaches after courses of acupuncture treatment or chiropractic spinal alignment. These modalities are safe and at times extremely effective, so they should be considered along with the treatments described above.

Young women are often susceptible to frequent severe migraine headaches despite careful dietary manipulation and avoidance of possible precipitating factors. For them, using the drug propranolol (Inderal) may provide dramatic relief. However, because this is primarily an anti-hypertension drug, blood pres-

sure should be monitored frequently. Propranolol should be
slowly discontinued prior to anesthesia and major surgery.
Also, be aware that it does cross the placenta, and studies have
not yet determined whether or not it is toxic to a developing
fetus. Low concentrations of propanolol may be excreted
breast milk. And it may cause elevation of blood cholesterol.
The good news for young women is that their migraines typically disappear after several years. Therefore, it's a good idea
to slowly reduce the dosage of Inderal every six months to a
year, in hopes that the problem will be outgrown and the medication will no longer be required.

One new medication recently introduced for the treatment of
migraine headaches is Imitrex (sumatriptan), a prescription
drug presently available only in an injectable form. Patients
receive an automated syringe device and when they feel a headache coming on simply inject themselves with this powerful
drug. Imitrex is being heavily marketed and may prove beneficial for patients suffering from intractable migraine headaches. However, each dosage costs about $30 and there can
be dangerous side effects, such as severe disturbances of the
heart rhythm, dizziness, and blood pressure elevation. I have
prescribed this medication for several patients, but have done
so reluctantly.

I personally believe it is more appropriate to diligently work
to identify the underlying *causes* of migraine headaches, and
eliminate them, rather than simply treating the symptoms with
powerful medications.

LifeGuide

Recommendations

1. Identify and eliminate the following food additives from your diet: Aspartame (NutraSweet), monosodium glutamate (MSG), sulfites and nitrates.

2. Eliminate caffeine (totally) from your diet. Read food and medications labels to discern hidden sources of caffeine.

3. Stop smoking. If you don't smoke, avoid second-hand smoke.

4. Visit an optometrist for a routine eye examination.

5. Avoid tyramine-containing foods such as yogurt, liver, vinegar, yeast extracts, alcohol (especially red wine and champagne), chocolate, cheese and citrus fruits.

6. Try a food-elimination program (as described in this chapter).

7. Engage in some form of aerobic, low-impact exercise at least five times each week.

8. Seek ways to reduce stress. Investigate biofeedback or hypnotherapy. Learn a meditation technique.

9. Try taking the herb *feverfew* (1 capsule, 3 times per day for 3 to 4 weeks).

10. Supplement your diet with a good source of omega-3 fatty acids. I recommend 1-2 tablespoons of fresh cold-pressed flaxseed oil each day. This may cause some loosening of the stool for the first 1 to 2 weeks. Omega-6 fatty acids are also extremely helpful. Try taking four to five capsules of evening primrose oil each day.

11. Stop using perfume or cologne for four to six weeks.

12. Keep a headache diary to help identify situations, foods, or other possible triggers and assist in measuring your progress.

13. Take vitamin E (Carlson brand) 100 IU each day if you are hypertensive—if not, 400 IU each day (with food).

RESOURCES

1. For more information regarding diet and headache write to the National Headache Foundation, 5252 N. Western Ave., Chicago, IL 60625.

2. I recommend reading *Eighteen Natural Ways to Beat A Headache* by Norman D. Ford (Keats Publishing, Inc. New Canaan, CT: 1990). This is a terrific paperback reference book full of wonderful techniques, each of which may prove to be beneficial for your particular headache problem.

REFERENCES

1. Stewart, W.F., et al. Prevalence of migraine headache. JAMA. Jan. 1, 1992; Vol. 267; No. 1. pp. 64-69.

2. Hampton, Nell. "Heading off headache." Vegetarian Times. March 1992. pp. 58-64.

3. Lipton, R.B., Newman, L.C., et al. "Aspartame as a dietary trigger of headache." Headache. 29: 90-92. 1989.

4. Manahan, William. Eat For Health. H.J. Cramer, Inc. publisher. Tiburon, CA. 1988. pp. 101-105.

5. Hughes, E.C., et al. "Migraine: A diagnostic test for etiology of food sensitivity by a nutritionally supported fast and confirmed by long-term report." Annals of Allergy. 55: 28-32. 1985.

6. Egger, J., et al. "Is migraine food allergy? A double-blind controlled trial of oligoantigenic diet treatment." Lancet. October 15, 1983. pp. 865-9.

7. Glueck, Charles. U. of Cincinnati College of Medicine-1986.

8. Hitzemann, R.J., Associate Professor of Psychiatry and Behavioral Sciences. State U. of NY. at Stoney-brook -1986.

9. Johnson, E.S., et al. "Efficacy of feverfew as prophylactic treatment of migraine." Brit. Med. J. 291: 569-73. 1985.

10. Mahaja, A.N.; Bailey, J.M. A platelet phospholipase inhibitor from the medicinal herb feverfew (tan-nacetum parthenium). Prostaglandins, Leukotrienes and Med. 8: 653-60. 1982.

15

Multiple Sclerosis:
The *LifeGuide* Plan

Nutritional and Lifestyle
Changes Can Help

Multiple sclerosis can be described as a disease modern society. It is far more common in geographic areas where populations consume high fat and highly processed foods as compared to those populations eating more fruits, vegetables and proteins derived from plant sources. For example, the incidence of multiple sclerosis is 6 to 14 per 100,000 in the southern United States and southern Europe and progressively increases to 30 to 80 per 100,000 in the northern United States, northern Europe and Canada. This striking geographic distribution of multiple sclerosis has long been known by research

scientists but has never really been pursued. Often explanations such as "an environmental factor" or "a virus" are offered
in textbooks, but these explanations are not substantiated by
any meaningful research.

A close examination of the incidence of multiple sclerosis
around the world reveals however that there are some areas in
northern latitudes that actually have very few cases of multiple
sclerosis. Countries like China, Japan and Korea, which are at a
similar latitude as the United States, have far fewer cases of MS.
Interestingly, the incidence of multiple sclerosis in Norway var-
ies quite dramatically from one district to another.

Roy L. Swank, M.D., provided one key to this puzzle when
he published research in 1952 showing a direct correlation between the incidence of multiple sclerosis in various districts
of Norway and the amount of dietary fat consumed in those
specific areas.[1] This important but largely unrecognized discovery offers the most meaningful explanation about why MS
is so common in some areas and almost unknown in others.
People in countries like Japan, Korea and China have until
recently, consumed diets far lower in fat than those in countries with high rates of MS like the United States, Canada and
most of northern Europe. Although several studies have confirmed Swank's original hypothesis, the concept that nutrition
plays any significant role in multiple sclerosis has not gained
a strong foothold in modern western medical thinking.[2,3]

Multiple sclerosis, like many other diseases of modern civilization, is caused by an overactive and misdirected immune system. For reasons that are unclear, the immune system reacts
against the protective insulating cover (myelin) of the nerves

of the central nervous system (the brain and spinal cord). White blood cells called lymphocytes attack myelin as if it were an invading organism or foreign substance. When the body's immune system fails to control itself and lymphocytes attack normal body tissues, the disease process that ensues is called an autoimmune disease. Other autoimmune diseases include: rheumatoid arthritis, systemic lupus erythematosus (SLE) and even some forms of vascular disease.

The typical western medical response to these autoimmune diseases, including multiple sclerosis, is to administer potent medicines designed to turn off the over activity of the immune system that characterizes these illnesses. Unfortunately, these potent immunosuppressant drugs, such as cortisone, Prednisone, Methotrexate and Cytoxan, reduce the effectiveness of the entire immune system and are fraught with other life-threatening side effects.

Somehow, in cases of multiple sclerosis, the lymphocytes get their signals crossed. It's as if they receive a message directing them to attack the brain and spinal cord. But what are the messages that control lymphocytes? Lymphocytes receive direction from a group of chemicals called *prostaglandins*, so named because they were first isolated from the prostate gland. Prostaglandins can be conveniently divided into three main groups, PG 1, PG 2 and PG 3, each of which is derived from a special type of dietary fats called the *essential fatty acids*. These special fats are not produced in the human body. They are called essential because without them we couldn't survive. The two essential fatty acids which lead to the production of prostaglandins are linolenic acid and linoleic acid, also known as omega 3 and omega 6 fatty acids, respectively.

The role of prostaglandins 1 and 3 is to moderate the immune response. Prostaglandins in group 2, on the other hand, signal the lymphocytes to become more active in the immune response. In normal situations a balance is achieved. Under the influence of prostaglandin 2 the white blood cells are activated, but this activity is kept from getting out of hand by prostaglandins from groups 1 and 3. Interestingly, in people suffering from multiple sclerosis, the cerebrospinal fluid has been shown to contain significantly less linoleic acid than in non-afflicted individuals. Linoleic acid is the precursor to prostaglandin 1. Prostaglandin 3 is derived from linolenic acid.

What emerges from this simplified understanding of immune function is that it is possible for MS patients to *naturally* gain more control over their condition. This is easily done by increasing dietary intake of linoleic and linolenic acids, which will stimulate the production of more "good prostaglandins," from groups 1 and 3.

This approach to the treatment of multiple sclerosis has been followed for decades in Europe and Scandinavian countries. Researchers like Dr. Jan DeVries have long supported the use of essential fatty acid supplementation products not only to treat the symptoms of multiple sclerosis, but also to reduce the frequency of new episodes.

Any multiple sclerosis sufferer who has spent time exploring non-mainstream approaches, has likely discovered frequent references to *evening primrose oil*. Used by native American Indians for a variety of skin conditions and infections, the healing power of evening primrose has been known for centuries. Over the past half century this special plant oil has been widely recommended in Europe as a nutritional supplement for the treatment of multiple sclerosis.

What is it about evening primrose oil that makes it so useful in treating multiple sclerosis? Analysis reveals that it is a very rich source of linoleic acid, the essential fatty acid that serves as the precursor to prostaglandin 1 which is critically important in controlling the immune system. Another rich source of linoleic acid is borage oil. These two supplements are now widely available in health food stores.

Prostaglandin 3, although much less potent than prostaglandin 1, nevertheless plays an important role in that it reduces the production of the dangerous prostaglandin 2. Prostaglandin 3 is derived from the other essential fatty acid, linolenic acid, which can also be supplemented in the diet. One excellent source is flaxseed oil which is more that 50 linolenic acid.

There are certain dietary factors that lead to the production of prostaglandin 2 and so likely worsen symptoms of multiple sclerosis. Perhaps the biggest trigger of prostaglandin 2 production is dietary fat, especially saturated fats and cholesterol. Alcohol also leads to the production of prostaglandin 2. Prostaglandin 2 is diminished by a diet rich in zinc, vitamin C, vitamins B^3 and B^6 and linolenic acid.

It is clear that a low-fat diet is critical for multiple sclerosis sufferers. In one 17-year study, of 146 patients who adopted very low-fat diets, multiple sclerosis progressed much less rapidly than in patients on normal diets. In addition, there was a significant reduction in the death rate among those on the low-fat diet. As Dr. Swank indicated, "If treated early in the disease, before significant disability had developed, a high percentage of cases remain unchanged for up to 20 years."[4]

Nutritionists, naturopaths, chiropractors and holistically oriented medical doctors have for years been treating multiple sclerosis with essential fatty acid supplements, vitamins and minerals fat-restricted diets, with *great success*. This approach is based on strengthening the body and working with nature — rather than fighting a war using potent immunosuppressive drugs, where the patient becomes the battlefield.

Clearly, modern immunosuppressive medicines may at times have a role in the treatment of acute and severe symptoms of multiple sclerosis, but they should not be relied upon in an attempt to maintain good health.

In the late 1950's and early 1960's researchers in England began exploring some interesting similarities between MS and deficiency of vitamin B_{12}. They noted that pernicious anemia, a type of anemia caused by low levels of vitamin B_{12}, like MS, is much more prevalent in Northern Europe as compared to Southern Europe and tropical areas. More recent studies have revealed that patients suffering from MS very frequently have red blood cells which are larger than those of the normal population, much like patients suffering from vitamin B_{12} deficiency[5]. In fact, in a study recently completed at King's College in England, it was noted that a large proportion of patients suffering from MS had lower blood levels of vitamin B_{12} when compared to normal control groups[6]. But the possible connection between MS and vitamin B_{12} deficiency is even more profound. Vitamin B_{12} deficiency in and of itself leads to significant problems of the nervous system. Specifically, in the absence of adequate amounts of vitamin B_{12} various parts of the nervous system experience destruction of the myelin covering over nerves similar to that which occurs in MS. This is because vitamin B_{12} plays an integral role in the formation and maintenance of healthy myelin[7]. Some researchers believe that a low level of vitamin B_{12} because of its effect on regulation of the immune system, may make some patients more vulnerable to a certain virus which may be responsible for MS[8]. Regardless of the mechanism involved in the relationship between a low vitamin B_{12} level and MS, the importance of adequate levels of vitamin B_{12} in the maintenance of healthy myelin as well as its role in stabilizing the immune response provides clear justification of its use as a supplement in multiple sclerosis. I frequently teach my MS patients how to administer B_{12} by intramuscular injection in a dosage of approximately 1,000 mcg. (1 cc.) once or twice each month. During an acute MS flare-up, I typically administer 1,000 mcg. (1 cc.) by injection intramuscularly each day for a ten to fourteen day period. Obviously, it makes sense to monitor the B_{12} level. A serum B_{12} level is a simple and inexpensive blood test. Normal values are between 232-1138 pg/ml. I try to keep my patients' levels in the high therapeutic range (900-1100).

With proper attention to diet and lifestyle, as well as the use of effective nutritional supplements, multiple sclerosis is almost always easily brought under control and the body harmonized.

LifeGuide

RECOMMENDATIONS

1. Reduce dietary fat immediately and significantly. Total fat should be no more than 18 percent of total calories.

2. Use essential fatty acid supplementation. Try one and eventually two tablespoons of fresh flaxseed oil and two to three capsules of evening primrose oil or borage oil each day. These supplements are widely available at health food stores.

3. Eliminate consumption of cholesterol, saturated fats and alcohol. Without question the best diet for multiple sclerosis is *totally* vegetarian.

4. Add vitamin C (Ester C with bioflavonoids), 3,000-5,000 milligrams each day.

5. Add vitamin B-Complex with vitamin B_{12}, 50 milligrams twice a day.

6. Take a multi-mineral supplement supplying 50 milligrams of zinc each day.

7. Take vitamin E (Carlson brand) 100 IU each day if you are hypertensive—if not, 400 IU each day (with food).

8. Avoid exposure to heat. Stay out of hot tubs and sauna baths, and avoid becoming overheated when exercising.

9. Learn a meditation or relaxation technique and practice it regularly. Regular meditation has been shown to be effective in other autoimmune diseases and will very likely benefit MS patients.

10. Have your doctor check your vitamin B_{12} level.

11. Take Pycnogenol 50 mg. each day. This is a potent antioxidant which readily enters the brain and spinal cord.

RESOURCES

1. I recommend reading *Multiple Sclerosis* by Dr. Jan DeVries (Mainstream Publishing Company, Edin-burgh). This very informative book can usually be found in health food stores and contains very useful information, not only about nutritional considerations in multiple sclerosis but also information about hyperbaric oxygen, homeopathy, acupuncture, dental care and enzyme therapy.

2. Other information about multiple sclerosis can be obtain by contacting MULTIPLE SCLEROSIS NATIONAL SOCIETY, 205 East 42nd Street, Manhattan, NY, 10017. (212) 986-3240, or contact the Multiple Sclerosis Foundation, Inc., at 1-800-441-7055.

REFERENCES

1. Swank, R.L., Lerstad, O., Strom, A., et al: Multiple sclerosis in rural
    Norway: Its geographical and occupational incidence in relation to nu-
    trition. NewEngJMed. Vol. 246: 721-728, 1952.
2. Agranoff, W.B., Goldberg, David: Diet and the geographic distribution
    of multiple sclerosis. Lancet. Nov. 2, 1974. pp. 1061-66.
3. Alter, M., Yamoor, M., Harshe, M.: Multiple sclerosis and nutrition.
    ArchNeurol. Vol. 31: Oct. 1974. pp. 267-72.
4. Swank, R.L.: Multiple sclerosis: 20 years on low-fat diet. ArchNeurol.
    Vol. 23: Nov. 1974. 60-74.

16

Lou Gehrig's Disease

Progress in the Treatment of Amyotrophic Lateral Sclerosis

Amyotrophic lateral sclerosis (ALS), also known as Lou Gehrig's disease, is typically described as a universally fatal, hopeless affliction, for which there is no cure. Indeed, most textbooks on the subject indicate that this disease progresses to death in a matter of two to six years after the diagnosis has been made.

Although ALS has been described in medical textbooks dating back to the middle of the nineteenth century, very little has ever been learned about the actual cause of this affliction until now.

A recent editorial appearing in the British medical journal, *The*

Lancet, reported, "There is also evidence that mortality from the disease is changing rapidly over time. Death rates from motoneuron disease (ALS) have increased at all ages over the past two decades in the USA, the UK, and Scandinavia. Although there is still some uncertainty about the true magnitude of the increase, there can be little doubt that motoneuron disease (ALS) has become more common in the countries of the Western world." Further, this editorial indicated that "... some factor associated with "westernization" influences the risk of getting the disease."[1] So ALS, like atherosclerosis, most forms of cancer, osteoporosis, multiple sclerosis, Alzheimer's disease, arthritis, and hypercholesterolemia, can clearly be characterized as "an illness created by modern man." But what is it about our modern Western society that is leading to ever increasing rates of these and other diseases? As I have already pointed out in earlier chapters, there is no question that the nutritional changes that have taken place over the past century, particularly with respect to fat consumption, have had a profound effect on the regulation of our immune systems. In addition, we are now learning that a wide array of modern day maladies are caused by "free radical damage."

"Free radicals" is a term used to describe several types of oxygen atoms normally produced within our bodies during the course of cellular metabolism. Free radicals are used by the body to destroy harmful bacteria and viruses and are also involved in the production of hormones, carrying chemical messages, and in the activitization of various enzyme systems. When the immune system is overactive, as is the case in most "modern diseases," excessive amounts of free radicals are produced which damages healthy tissue. Excess free radicals are also produced when our bodies are exposed to toxic waste, radiation, air pollution, tobacco smoke, and pesticides.

This is the reason that most nutritionally-minded healthcare practitioners recommend a group of vitamins and minerals called "antioxidants" since these supplements limit the life span of free radicals and therefore can reduce the damaging effects that our modern environment and diet have upon our health.

Fascinating new research from the Massachusetts General Hospital in Boston has recently revealed that many cases of ALS are, in fact, caused by a deficiency of an enzyme which normally reduces the life span of free radicals in the central nervous system[2]. This antioxidant enzyme, known as super-oxide dismutase (SOD), has long been studied as a possible missing link in the biochemistry of cancer cells since it is known that SOD levels are highly diminished during malignancy. It has also been noted that SOD has been used to protect normal tissue from damage by ionizing radiation and, by limiting the cellular damage caused by free radicals, SOD may be directly involved in the control of the aging process[3].

The importance of the discovery of the relationship between deficiencies of SOD and amyotrophic lateral sclerosis is two-fold. First, it confirms what scientists have long suspected about this and other degenerative diseases of the central nervous system as being related to simply an uncontrolled advanced rate of aging. Secondly, this fundamental understanding of the mechanism of tissue destruction in ALS gives strong support to a program which not only enhances the body's ability to produce SOD, but also provides other powerful antioxidants designed to limit the life span of tissue-destroying free radicals.

Unfortunately, because SOD is a small protein molecule which is broken down during the process of digestion, efforts to increase the body's SOD activity with oral supplementation of this enzyme have been unsuccessful. However, it may be possible to increase the body's SOD activity by supplying increased amounts of the raw materials necessary for its production. These nutrients include copper, zinc, and, to a lesser extent, manganese. In a study performed at the University of Utah College of Medicine, researchers found that experimental animals given a diet deficient in copper demonstrated significantly decreased SOD activity in body tissues[3]. In another study performed at the University of Wisconsin, supplementation of manganese in humans was found to significantly increase blood levels of SOD[3].

Obviously, it makes sense to add dietary antioxidants such as vitamins C, E, and beta carotene. But, unfortunately, the central nervous system tends to exclude these potent antioxidants from its domain. The gatekeeper between the blood and the actual tissue of the central nervous system is known "blood-brain barrier." Because of the brain's profound sensitivity and strict requirements, the blood-brain barrier is permeable only to a small number of molecules and chemicals—allowing them passage to the sanctuary of the brain and spinal cord.

Fortunately, a very potent antioxidant is available which has the unique characteristic of being able to penetrate the blood-brain barrier with ease. This naturally derived antioxidant, Pycnogenol, is derived from the bark of the maritime pine tree which grows along the coast of Europe from southern France to the Spanish border. Pycnogenol has been reported to be as much as 50 times more potent than vitamin E and 20 times stronger that vitamin C with respect to its antioxidant capabilities and may, in fact, be the most powerful naturally occurring antioxidant known[3]. Fortunately, Pycnogenol is widely available in health food stores and does not require a doctor's prescription.

Research from the Mt. Sinai School of Medicine published in The Lancet in 1988 revealed that ALS patients whose diets were supplemented with an amino acid preparation containing high levels of the amino acids L-leucine, L-isoleucine, and L-valine demonstrated significant benefit in terms of maintaining the strength of their arms and legs and ability to continue walking. These supplements were chosen because it was hypothesized that some patients with ALS had a deficiency of a certain enzyme which could be stimulated with these particular amino acid. These amino acids are typically available at most health food stores or they may be ordered from MetaMetrix Laboratories (see References). In the study, subjects consumed three grams of L-leucine, two grams of L-isoleucine, and 1.6 grams of L-valine four times daily between meals[4].

Finally, perhaps one of the most exciting prospects in the treatment of amyotrophic lateral sclerosis is the use of dehydroepiandrosterone (DHEA). DHEA is a naturally occurring steroid produced in the adrenal glands. It typically reaches its peak level at approximately age 20 and then declines progressively with age to the extent that by age 80 blood levels of DHEA are reduced to only about 5 percent of what they were at age 20 [5]. Dr. Alan Gaby writing in Holistic Medicine reveals that DHEA may be of value in preventing and treating a wide range of medical problems including high cholesterol, cardiovascular disease, diabetes, cancer, Alzheimer's disease, immune system disorders, chronic fatigue, and AIDS[6]. The mechanism by which DHEA exerts its powerful influence is not clear, but it has been described as an "anti-aging hormone," and it is likely for this reason that it has been tried and found effective for such a wide variety of ailments.

In a recent issue of The Townsend Letter for Doctors, Dr. Gaby reported the case of a 78-year-old man with a six-year history of progressive neurologic deterioration as a consequence of ALS. His serum DHEA level was found to be in the low normal range. The patient was started on oral supplemental DHEA and over a period of two months, there was a dramatic improvement in his swallowing ability, his appetite, and his general well being.

Recently a 68-year-old woman suffering from ALS came under my care. Her condition had deteriorated to the extent that her speech and swallowing were moderately affected and she was wheelchair bound. I began treatment with 50 mg. of DHEA by mouth every other day. At her first follow-up visit one month after starting DHEA she was able to stand and take several steps for the first time in six months. As of this writing, her situation has not significantly deteriorated, although I have not noted any continued improvement. She is presently taking 50 mg. of DHEA each day.

DHEA is safe and inexpensive. Unfortunately, it is available only by prescription and to my knowledge from only two pharmacies in this country. (See References).

Although these recommendations do not specifically offer a cure for ALS, because of their sound scientific support they do at least offer help—and that may be the most potent medicine of all.

LifeGuide
RECOMMENDATIONS

1. Take the following minerals to enhance production of su-
    peroxide dismutase (SOD):
    - zinc (glycine, histidine dipeptide chelate) 5 mg.
    - copper (lysine dipeptide chelate) 500 mcg.
    - manganese (glycine dipeptide chelate) 2 mg.
    These micronutrients should be taken each day.

2. Take relatively high dosages of vitamin antioxidants including:
    - ascorbate powder, 2,000 mg. three times a day
    - vitamin E (natural) 400 IU, increasing to 1,000 IU over
      three to four weeks with food each day
    - beta carotene 25,000 IU each day with food.
    Because of its antioxidant properties, take selenium 100-150
    mcg. each day.

4. Pycnogenol. This powerful antioxidant is available at most
    health food stores. Start with 50 mg. each day and after two
    to three weeks increase to 100 mg. each day.

5. Take the following amino acids four times each day between
    meals:
    - L-leucine, 3 grams
    - L-isoleucine, 2 grams
    - L-valine, 1.6 grams
    If these are unavailable at your health food outlet, contact
    MetaMetrix Medical Laboratories at:
    5000 Peachtree Indus. Blvd., #110
    Norcross, GA 30071
    (404) 446-5483

LifeGuide
RECOMMENDATIONS

(continued)

6.   DHEA. Begin with 50 mg. every other day and after two
     to three weeks increase to 50 mg. each day. Dosages as
     high as 100 mg. each day may be given under the direc-
     tion of a physician. DHEA is available from:
          Belmar Pharmacy
          8015 West Alameda Avenue, Suite 100
          Lakewood, CO 80226.
          (800) 525-9473
                    or try:
          College Pharmacy
          833 N Tejon Street
          Colorado Springs, CO 80903
          (800) 748-2263

RESOURCES

1   ALS and Neuromuscular Research Foundation
     Pacific Presbyterian Medical Center
     2351 Clay Street, #416
     San Francisco, CA 94115
     (415) 923-3604

2.   National ALS Association
     15300 Ventura Boulevard, Suite 315
     Sherman Oaks, CA 91403
     (818) 990-2151

For more information on Pycnogenol, read The New Superantioxidant-Plus, by Richard A. Passwater, Ph.D., (Keats Publishing, Inc., New Canaan, CT). This small paperback monograph is available at most health food stores and gives a thorough understanding of the usefulness of this very potent antioxidant.

REFERENCES

1.   The Lancet, Volume 336, October 27, 1990, pp. 1033-34.
2.   Rosen, D., Siddique, T., et al, Mutations in the Cu/Zn Superoxide Dismutase Gene are Associated with Familial Amyotrophic Lateral Sclerosis. Nature Volume 362, March 4, 1993, pp. 59-62.
3.   Life Extenders and Memory Boosters, David Steinman, Editor, Health Quest Publications, Reno, Nevada, 1993.
4.   Plaitakis, A., Mandeli, J., et al, Pilot Trial of Branched-Chain Amino Acids in Amyotrophic Lateral Sclerosis, Lancet, May 7, 1988, pp. 1015-1018.
5.   Whitaker, Julian. Health and Healing - Tomorrow's Medicine Today. June 1992.
6.   Gaby, A., DHEA: The Hormone That "Does it All," Holistic Medicine, Spring 1993, pp. 19-23.

17

Herbs and Health
A Modern Role for
Ancient Wisdom

Most people would be surprised if their doctors recommended herbs for their medical problems. They might also be surprised to learn that in the United States today approximately 25 percent of all prescription drugs contain active ingredients derived from plants. Some examples are shown in Table 2 on the following page.

Drug	Herb	Use
Donnatal	*Belladonna*	Reduces spasm of digestive tract.
Lanoxin	*Foxglove*	Regulates heart rhythm.
Reserpine	*Snakeroot*	Reduces high blood pressure.
Theo-Dur	*Thea*	Reduces bron- chial spasms.
Senokot	*Senna*	Laxative

The use of herbs for treating illness and sustaining health was first recorded 5,000 years ago. Chinese physicians used *ma huang*, also known as Chinese ephedra, for bronchial conges- tion, colds and asthma. One of ephedra's active ingredients, *pseudoephedrine*, is contained in many over-the-counter cold remedies including Sudafed, (which derives its name from this herb). The World Health Organization estimates that two- thirds of the world's population, about four billion people, rely primarily on herbs for medical problems.[1]

During the past several decades, Americans have shown an increasing interest in healing herbs. We seem to be taking a greater interest in self-care, and healing herbs naturally compliment lifestyles centered around sound nutrition, preventive medicine and overall fitness. We are also beginning to recognize that significant dangers are associated with some "pharmaceutical advances." For example, the FDA's restriction on silicone breast implants and the recently disclosed health risks of the sleeping pill Halcion, have helped encourage the search for safer and more natural alternatives.

Americans are becoming acutely aware that the greatest resource for combating disease is Mother Nature. The National Cancer Institute has investigated more than 70,000 plant extracts and has found antitumor properties in more than 10 percent.[2] Taxol, derived from the bark of the Pacific Yew Tree, shows significant promise in the treatment of ovarian and other cancers. Vincristine, an extremely potent anticancer agent, is derived from the Madagascar Periwinkle. Events such as these have helped us rediscover the potential that nature offers in the treatment of disease. As important as such rediscoveries are, their continuation could be in jeopardy. About 140 species of plants and animals become extinct *every day,* and in light of thier potential healing powers, a new sense of urgency is added to efforts to reduce our impact on the environment.

It is not surprising that in developed societies physicians rarely use herbs. Every day doctors are bombarded by literature promoting the latest drugs. Representatives of the large pharmaceutical companies visit physicians almost daily to push their company's products. Most doctor's offices have large "drug closets" where these representatives leave free samples which physicians, in turn, distribute to patients.

Healing herbs, on the other hand, are not heavily promoted. Since they cannot be patented, the profits in packaging and distributing them are minuscule compared with the huge profits from synthetic drugs.

In addition, because many herbal preparations require a period of time to produce positive results, the "quick fix" sought by many patients is not available. In efforts to please their patients, some physicians have a tendency to prescribe remedies that alleviate the immediate symptoms, without attempting to uncover the underlying causes of illness.

The modern physician's reliance upon laboratory-developed pharmaceuticals is one manifestation of a society that places its complete trust in science and technology. As author Marti Kheel explains, "Rather than use the entire plant, western medicine prefers to isolate the plant's most active ingredients in order to develop a more potent force. However, in general, isolated and 'refined' drugs are much more toxic than are the substances from which they are derived. (It is no coincidence that the word *pharmaceutical* derives from an ancient Greek word meaning 'poison.')"[3]

Having never been formally trained in the therapeutic use of herbs, I frequently rely on texts that provide information about which herbs are helpful in a particular situation and also what precautions should be taken when using those herbs. While herbs are typically a much safer alternative than pharmaceutical drugs, *any* remedy, either herbal or pharmaceutical, can have side effects which must be understood. Some herbs for example should not be given during pregnancy. Others may react with other herbs or prescription drugs, causing dangerous side effects. Of the hundreds of healing herbs available, there are four that have had such an impact on my medical practice that I utilize them virtually every day: feverfew, garlic, ginger and echinacea.

FEVERFEW

As a neurologist, I have had great success prescribing the herb feverfew for many patients who suffer from intractable headaches. If a patient has been diligent in attempting to identify and eliminate dietary and environmental headache "triggers," I will prescribe one capsule of feverfew, three times a day. Frequently this leads to a reduction not only of the intensity but also the frequency of headaches. I have also found feverfew to be helpful in relieving chronic pain in conditions such as arthritis and low back disorders.

GARLIC

I regularly include garlic in nutritional programs I created for patients with such problems as hypertension, high cholesterol, respiratory infections and strokes. The value of garlic in treating medical problems has been known for thousands of years. The builders of the pyramids ate garlic daily to increase endurance and strength. Its attributes have been described in the Bible as well as in ancient Hebrew, Greek and Roman literature.

Toward the end of the 19th century, doctors noted remarkably high cure rates among tuberculosis patients who were treated with garlic. During World War I garlic was often used to treat wounds and infections and to prevent gangrene. It became known as "Russian penicillin" because of its widespread use in that country.

Many well-controlled scientific studies have shown that garlic has significant antibacterial activity against numerous strains of harmful bacteria.[4-6] In addition, garlic has significant antifungal activity against *Candida Albicans*, the organism that causes most cases of vaginal yeast infection.[7] In 1973, the *Japanese Journal of the Association for Infectious Diseases* published the results of a large well-controlled study which proved the effectiveness of garlic against influenza.[8]

The beneficial properties of garlic are primarily due to a substance called *allicin* which is activated when garlic is chewed or cut. In addition to allicin, garlic contains vitamins A, B^1, B^2 and C, as well as zinc, selenium, calcium, germanium, iron and magnesium. Obviously, this is more than just a "folk remedy." Fortunately, in order to reap its benefits, you don't have to risk the alienation of friends and family by chewing several cloves of garlic each day. Preparations like Kyolic® provide the beneficial properties of garlic without the pungent odor and taste are readily available. However, it is highly desirable to use fresh garlic whenever appropriate in cooking. To measure the effectiveness of garlic preparations, determine how much allicin (garlic's active ingredient) they contain. Try to consume approximately 1,500 to 2,000 micrograms of allicin each day. Fortunately, commercial preparations of garlic are fairly inexpensive—about $8 to $12 for a month's supply.

GINGER

Ginger ale has long been used to relieve upset stomachs, nausea and other digestion problems. This common folk remedy has its roots in ancient medical lore dating back to around 3,000 B.C. Ancient Chinese texts describe the usefulness of ginger for menstrual cramps, arthritis and seasickness. A recent study reported in the prestigious British medical journal, *The Lancet*, showed that ginger root was significantly better in preventing motion sickness than an over-the-counter drug, Dramamine.[9] Other studies have shown that ginger root is effective for nausea caused by car, boat, train, and plane travel. Other medical problems that may be alleviated by ginger include: menstrual cramps, colds and flu, arthritis and high cholesterol.

Available at most grocery stores, ginger root is used to make the powder in ginger capsules. The root can be grated and made into ginger tea, which is helpful for a variety of medical problems. It may, however, cause "heartburn," in which case the dosage should be reduced or eliminated completely. For motion sickness I recommend taking two or four capsules of ginger powder an hour before starting a trip. An additional one or two capsules can be taken every two hours as needed. For colds with congestion, try three to four tablespoons of fresh ginger juice in a warm bath.

ECHINACEA

Echinacea, also known as the Purple Cone Flower, has been a favorite herbal remedy in this country for centuries. From the 1890s until the mid-1920s, extracts from the root of the echinacea plant were commonly used for a variety of medical problems. Unfortunately, its popularity diminished in the 1930s as antibiotics became more widely available. Today, echinacea is virtually unknown to American doctors, although in Europe it continues to be widely recommended.

Echinacea is useful in treating arthritis as well as in the healing of wounds. Perhaps its most common use is in prevention and treatment of the common cold. Andrew Weil, M.D., in his book, *Natural Health, Natural Medicine*, recommends using echinacea "as a first line of treatment for common infections before resorting to conventional antibiotics. Use it for colds, flu, sore throats and episodes of low resistance." Weil indicates that echinacea losses its usefulness when taken on a continual basis for more than two weeks at a time.

Echinacea, available at health food stores, comes in a variety of forms including capsules, tinctures and extracts. Since echinacea should produce a numbing sensation when held in the mouth for a few minutes, this is a good way to determine its potency.

Extracts from the echinacea root have been the subject of more than 350 scientific studies worldwide. Laboratory testing has shown that these extracts increase the function of the immune system in a variety of ways. Not only does echinacea increase the number of immune system cells but it also increases their effectiveness in fighting disease.[10,11] Michael Castleman, in *The Healing Herbs*, reports that echinacea may be used by patients undergoing radiation therapy to reduce the chances of infection. He cautions patients, however, to consult with their doctors prior to using this herb.

Taking this time-proven herbal remedy at the onset of a cold is often surprisingly effective. I prefer using the tincture and recommend one full dropper in a small glass of water, three to four times a day for a week or two.

Although I've described only a few important herbs, there are hundreds available which are beneficial for treating various problems. Before using any herbal product, read about it in one of the many excellent herbal texts available. (See Resources.) Since herbal products do not require a prescription (at least not yet), they provide means for patients to take charge of their own health.

RESOURCES

1. *The Healing Herbs* by Michael Castleman (Rhodale Press. Emmaus, PA. 1991) is an extremely well written, user-friendly guide to the therapeutic use of herbs.

2. *The Scientific Validation of Herbal Medicine* by Daniel B. Mowry, Ph.D., (Cormorant Books, 1986) is a wonderfully annotated textbook describing the use of herbs, vitamins, minerals and other nutrients to treat specific medical problems.

3. *Let's Remedy the Situation* by Velma J. Keith and Monteen Gordon (Mayfield Publications. P.O. Box 157. Pleasant Grove, UT. 84062), is an easy-to-read herbal reference guide and "How To" herb book.

4. Natural Health, The Guide to Well-Being is a bi-monthly magazine with informative articles about healing herbs in almost every issue. It is available at many newsstands or can be ordered by calling: (800) 666-8576. Or write: EastWest Natural Health, Subscription Department, P.O. Box 52372, Boulder, CO 80323-2372.

5. In the monthly magazine, Vegetarian Times, you'll find The Herbalist, a department in each issue devoted to herbs. You can find Vegetarian Times in most book stores or call toll free: (800) 435-9610; (in Illinois call (800) 435-0715) or write: Vegetarian Times, P.O. Box 446, Mount Morris, IL 61054-9894.

REFERENCES

1. Castleman, Michael. *The Healing Herbs.* (Emmaus, PA. Rhodale Press) 1991. p. 1.

2. Ibid. p. 19.

3. Kheel, Marti. From healing herbs to deadly drugs western medicine's war against the natural world. Townsend Letter for Doctors. January 1992. p. 1-15.

4. Cavallito, C.J., et. al. The antibacterial principle of allium sativum. III. Its precursor and essential oil of garlic. Journal of the American Chemical Society. 67. 1032-1033. 1945.

5. Sharma, V.D., et. al. Antibacterial property of allium sativum Linn.: In vivo and in vetro studies. Indian Journal of Experimental Biology. 15 (6). 466-468. 1977.

6. Johnson, M.G., and Vaughn, R.H. Death of salmonella typhimurium and escherichia coli in the presence of freshly reconstituted dehydrated garlic and onion. Applied Microbiology. 17. 903-905. 1969.

7. Mowrey, Daniel B. *The Scientific Validation of Herbal Medicine.* (Cormorant Books). 1986. p. 122.

8. Nagai, K. Experimental studies on the preventive effect of garlic extract against infection with influence virus. Japanese Journal of the Association for Infectious Diseases. 47. 111-115. 1973.

9. Mowrey, D. B., and Clayson, D.E. Motion sickness, ginger and psychophysicis. The Lancet. March 20. 655-657. 1982.

10. Wagner, H. and Proksch, A. An immunostim-ulating active principle from Echinacea purpurea. A. Angew. Phytother. 2 (5). 166-178. 1981.

11. Op. cit. 1. p. 152.

18

Brain Tumors: Are You Talking Yourself to Death?

The Hidden Dangers of Hand-Held Cellular Telephones

"Our use of energy for power and communications has radically changed the total electromagnetic field of the Earth. Because we cannot directly perceive this with any of our senses, most of us are unaware that it has occurred. ...Today, we swim in a sea of energy that is almost totally man-made."

—Robert O. Becker, MD

Cross Currents.

In June of 1992, the United Nations Conference on Environment and Development was held in Rio de Janeiro. Representatives from 150 countries met at this "Earth Summit" to focus world-wide attention on a variety of environmental threats including air pollution, de-forestation, fresh water scarcity, soil erosion, acid rain and toxic waste. However, possibly because it isn't directly experienced by our senses—the dangers of electromagnetic radiation (EMR) received very little attention at this worldwide conference.

Electromagnetic radiation simply means energy transmission. Familiar examples of EMR include radio and television signals, visible light, ultra-violet light, microwave radio transmission, radar and X-rays.

Human beings have always been exposed to low levels of natural electromagnetic radiation. The sun produces various frequencies of visible and non-visible light and the earth itself produces a weak electromagnetic field as it rotates around its molten iron core. Humans have adapted well to this natural low-level background of EMR which has actually changed very little during the entire course of humanity—until just one century ago.

With the advent of the "electrical age," the electromagnetic environment to which humans had successfully adapted over millennia has been suddenly, dramatically and dangerously altered. We are now bombarded by a wide array of intense electromagnetic radiation from a variety of sources which have integrated their way into our day-to-day lives. We are exposed to dangerous microwave radiation from leaky microwave ovens and cellular telephones; we are blasted by radar whenever our speed is checked by a police radar gun or when we pass under an automatic door entering the grocery store; and we are almost constantly threatened by the so-called extremely low frequency (ELF) electromagnetic radiation produced by such commonly used devices as video display terminals, electric razors, television sets, hair dryers and electric blankets.

Power companies, cellular phone companies and electrical appliance manufacturers may report that these convenient, labor saving devices are perfectly safe. However, the truth of the matter is that exposure to these unnatural sources of EMR has definitely been shown to increase the risk of problems such as leukemia, brain cancer and birth defects.

A study published in 1979 showed that children living in homes where the wiring exposed them to high levels of EMR were 2-1/2 times more likely to die from leukemia than children exposed to normal levels of household electrical radiation. In addition, children with cancer were at least twice as likely to have lived near high current electrical power lines.[1] Research by Marjorie Speers of the University of Texas has clearly shown a profound increase in the incidence of brain tumors among those exposed to electromagnetic fields in the workplace. Incredibly, workers exposed to EMR in electric-power utilities were 13 *times* more likely to have brain tumors when compared to an unexposed comparison group.[2]

In another study, researchers investigating twenty-two cases of cancer among the staff of a California elementary school found that four pole-mounted electrical transformers were located just 10 feet away from the front of building. Interestingly, there were no cancer cases reported from those who worked in the back of the building.[3]

Living tissue is extremely sensitive to electromagnetic radiation and EMR is known to produce changes in the genetic components of living cells. According to Dr. Robert Becker, "Because abnormal electromagnetic fields can produce genetic abnormalities during cell division, it is quite possible that chronic exposure to such fields is a competent cause for the origin of cancer."[2]

Recently, a lawsuit was filed against a manufacturer of hand-held cellular phones by a man claiming that cellular phone use stimulated the development of a malignant brain tumor which took the life of his 33-year-old wife. Whether or not using that cellular phone led to this woman's brain tumor may never be known. But the important question raised by this complaint is the overall health risk hand-held cellular phones may pose for the roughly 3-4 million Americans who own them.

Unlike a new pharmaceutical drugs that must undergo rigorous safety evaluations for as long as seven years and often at a cost exceeding $200 million, no health safety evaluations were conducted on cellular phones before they were put on the market. Now that questions have been raised about the safety of these devices, the cellular industry is hastily issuing literature which they feel supports the safety of their products. In a recent publication by the cellular telecommunications industry association entitled, *CTIA White Paper on Electromagnetic Energy and Cellular Safety*, the cover page indicated that the document contained, "... unequivocal evidence that cellular phones are safe to use." However, no such evidence existed in the entire document. The document quoted a recent report from the Institute of Electrical and Electronics Engineers which, in fact, revealed that some cellular phones when held one centimeter or less from the head, actually caused higher levels of EMR exposure than allowed under International Radiation Protection Association guidelines.

Research to prove the safety of cellular telephones is simply not available. When commenting on the long-term carcinogenic effects of cellular phone usage, FDA's Chief of Radiation Biology Dr. Mays Swicord stated, "There's no reason at this point to suspect a problem, but I have to say we don't have a data base to clearly answer these questions."[4]

Fortunately, there has been considerable research exploring the dangers of exposure from such sources as radio transmitters, radar and microwave ovens. Cellular phones operate at a frequency similar to these sources of microwave radiation.

Research has shown an increase in the incidence of Down's syndrome in areas with large numbers of microwave transmitters and a much higher incidence of brain tumors among soldiers exposed to radar.[5] Researchers at the Medical College of Virginia have demonstrated a striking increase in the rate of proliferation of brain tumor cells after exposure to microwave radiation of the type used by cellular phones after just two hours.[6]

The dangers from microwave radiation of the frequencies emitted by cellular telephones have long been known by the military. In the *Military Standardization Handbook–Electromagnetic Radiation Hazards*, written August 10, 1973 and revised in 1983 this warning is given:

"The sensory elements of the body are located primarily in the skin tissues; for this reason, radiation frequencies below 1,000 MHz. are considered extremely hazardous because the presence EMR will not be detected by the human sensory system. Radiation at frequencies below 1,000 MHz. causes heat to be developed primarily in the deep tissues as a result of the penetration of the energy."

This means that the frequencies emitted by cellular telephones are doubly dangerous; not only will they cause heat in the deep tissues of the body; but this damage won't be felt by the victim.

Evidence supporting the dangers of microwave radiation is so compelling that staff researchers from the U.S. Environmental Protection Agency recommended that radio frequency and microwave radiation be designated a "possible carcinogen."[7]

Based on the accumulated evidence, it is obvious to many that hand-held cellular phones represent a significant health threat. Emanating high levels of EMR, these devices are held within a few inches of delicate brain tissue.[8]

Recently, a healthy, athletic 28-year-old man came to me after he suddenly collapsed while jogging. The brain scan revealed a small, malignant tumor on the surface of his brain exactly corresponding to the base of the antenna of his hand-held cellular telephone. (See figures 1 and 2.) He produced the owner's manual for his cellular telephone which contained this warning:

"DO NOT HOLD THE CELLULAR TELEPHONES SUCH THAT THE ANTENNA IS IN CONTACT WITH EXPOSED PARTS OF THE BODY, ESPECIALLY THE FACE OR EYES, WHILE THE UNIT IS TURNED ON."

If the cellular telephone industry believes, or would like us to believe, that their products are completely safe, *then why this warning?*

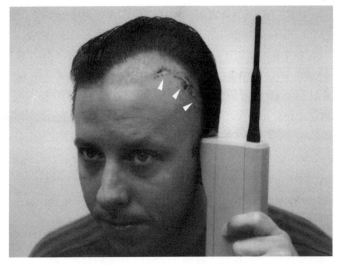

Figure 16-1 Matt Crist with hand-held Motorola Cellular Telephone. Note proximity of antenna to scar, indicated by arrows, from recent brain surgery

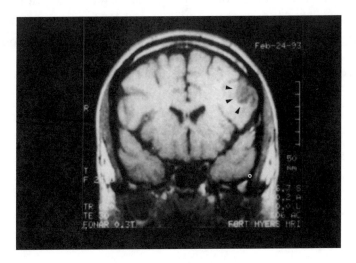

Figure 16-2 Matt Crist's MRI brain scan. Arrows indicate location of brain tumor.

Another patient, a 45-year-old real estate appraiser, recently underwent surgery to remove a large, highly malignant brain tumor from his right temporal lobe. (See figures 3 and 4.) This was followed by a full course of radiation therapy. He is, at the time of this writing, engaged in a course of potent intravenous chemotherapy. He purchased his NEC cellular telephone in November 1991, some seven months before his tumor was first diagnosed. He used this device regularly and did not make a connection between the hand-held cellular telephone and his brain tumor until he read this in the owner's manual:

"RADIO FREQUENCY INJURY: Your phone is a power transmitting device. When the phone is in use, radio frequency energy with a power output level ranging from 0.6 to 3.0 watts of radio frequency energy radiates from the antenna. Avoid direct contact with the phone antenna and/or direct exposure to the radio frequency energy radiated from the antenna at high level radiation periods."

Once again, I must ask, "*What does this mean?*" How can a person avoid exposure to the radio frequency energy, if these telephones transmit ten miles or more? It would appear that the reference to "high level radiation periods," means those times when the telephone is in use.

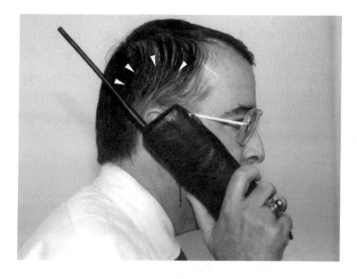

Figure 16-3 Bill Pogue demonstrating how he used his NEC hand-held cellular telephone. Arrows show location of brain tumor.

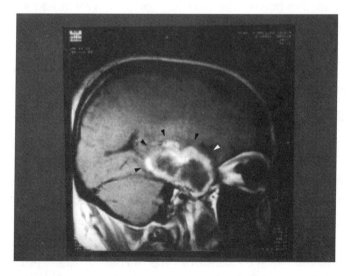

Figure 16-4 Bill Pogue's MRI brain scan. Arrows indicate location of highly malignant brain tumor.

In January 1993, these two patients and I traveled to New York where we met with Mr. David Reynard, the gentleman whose wife lost her battle with brain cancer. We first appeared on the *Faith Daniels Show* along with Ron Nessen, spokesperson for the cellular telephone industry, and Dr. Carl Sutton who has performed research dealing with the possible dangers of microwave radiation exposure.

During the program, Mr. Nessen made repeated attempts to assure the audience that hand-held cellular telephones were safe and that there were "thousands of research studies" available to prove his point. When challenged, he could produce only *one* research paper, a study written by the other guest on the program, Dr. Carl Sutton, entitled, *Studies of Long-Term Exposure of the Porcine Brain to Radiation from Two-Way Portable Radios.*[9]

Dr. Sutton's experiment, involved strapping radio transmitters to the heads of eight 200-pound pigs. The transmitters irradiated the pig's brains eight hours daily for a total of 90 days, after which Dr. Sutton executed the animals and examined their brains. The reports indicates that he did not find any "detectable brain injury."

What the cellular telephone industry neglected to tell us was that this experiment used radio transmitters operating at 452 MHz. which is *one-half* the frequency at which cellular telephones operate![9] We then decided to review other research conducted by the "medical expert" and found that he had published countless articles which described severe destruction to the brain and spinal cord in experimental animals subjected to microwave radiation. One of these studies, published in 1983, is called *Use of Non-Invasive Microwave Irradiation as a Spinal Cord Injury Model in Rats and Rabbits.*[10]

Following the *Faith Daniels* program, we appeared on ABC's *20/20*. During that appearance we reiterated the potential danger of hand-held cellular telephones. Coincidentally, that same day Craig McCaw, chairman of McCaw Cellular Communications, the nation's largest cellular telephone service company, announced his intention to commission a study of the potential dangers of this technology.

I cannot definitely prove that the brain tumors in my patients directly resulted from their use of cellular telephones, nor could I do so in other cases that are now surfacing all across the country. But the message is clear; EMR of the type given off by hand-held cellular telephones is dangerous. The cellular communications industry has misled the consumer into a false sense of security, much like the tobacco industry—which until just 30 years ago, was able to convince even a majority of physicians that cigarette smoking was safe.

The following are excerpts from a letter I submitted on February 3, 1993 to the New York Times, Washington Post, Chicago Tribune, Los Angeles Times, Miami Herald, Wall Street Journal, and many other major metropolitan newspapers.

URGENT

To The Editor:

With the recent concern surrounding the safety of hand-held cellular telephones, the cellular telephone communication industry has issued statements in an attempt to reassure the public that there are "thousands of studies" validating the safety of their product. Officials at the Environmental Protection agency (EPA) and the Food and Drug Administration (FDA), when challenged, have conceded that no such data exists.

The FDA, EPA and the cellular telephone communications industry have overlooked the existence of an extremely comprehensive long-term study which will surely either validate the safety of this product or condemn the industry. This study, presently ongoing, involves the use of some 3-4 million laboratory animals and is being conducted all across the United States. Over the next five to ten years, we will have ample data which will either substantiate or refute the assertions of the health risks posed by hand-held cellular telephones.

Unfortunately, the laboratory animals in this study are the millions of Americans who are currently using these devices. Unlike most other research endeavors, these test subjects have not provided informed consent to participate in this experiment.

On February 2, 1993, the FDA announced that it will require health hazard warning labels on all hand-held cellular telephones. Regardless of their motivation, it will be interesting to observe what effect this decision will have on the millions of Americans now the subjects of this grand experiment.

In the summer of 1993 I traveled to Chicago to testify as an expert witness in a class action suit brought against several of the large manufacturers of hand-held cellular telephones. During my testimony, the defense attorneys for the manufacturers of these devices asked me whether or not I was aware of the existence of any specific studies which would indicate that human electromagnetic exposure of the specific frequency given off by hand-held cellular telephone posed any health risk. My response, regardless of how many times they posed the question, was always the same—and that was that no specific studies of this type had been performed. They concluded, therefore, that this was an indication that their product was safe. I contend, however, that the complete absence of research represents a glaring error since research of frequencies above and below that used by cellular phones has clearly demonstrated a profound health risk. There are now some 4 million users of hand-held cellular telephones. According to the National Cancer Institute, the incidence of malignant brain tumors is approximately 8.5 per 100,000 adult population. That means that even if the use of these devices does not specifically cause brain tumors, each year there are an additional 400 Americans using hand-held cellular telephones who have brain tumors and don't know it. The scientific research clearly shows that these individuals are almost definitely accelerating the growth of their brain tumors and in so doing, directly shortening their life spans.

LifeGuide

RECOMMENDATIONS

1. Stop using hand-held portable cellular telephone.
2. Don't use an electric blanket
3. Don't sleep with a clock radio next to the head of your bed.
4. Avoid using electric razors, electric toothbrushes and blow-dryers.
5. Stay well back from television sets.
6. Stay at least three feet back from computer monitors.
7. Avoid using microwave ovens, or at least don't stand near when they are operating.
8. Do not live or work in a building that is near high tension electrical wires or transformers.
9. If your automobile has a rear window or trunk-mounted cellular telephone antenna, do not transmit or receive when passengers are in the rear seat.
10. If you have a transportable cellular telephone, keep the battery pack control unit as far as possible from your body.

RESOURCES

1. *Cross Currents* by Robert O. Becker, MD (Jeremy P. Tarcher, Inc., Los Angeles, CA, 1990). Dr. Becker's book not only describes the dangers of electro-pollution in our environment but also the future promise that electro-therapy may hold for health and healing.

2. *Currents of Death: Power Lines, Computer Terminals and the Attempts to Cover-up Their Threat to Your Health.* By P. Brodeur (Simon & Shuster, 1989).

3. *The Body Electric* by Robert O. Becker, MD and Gary Selden (William Morrow and Co., Inc., New York, New York, 1985). This is a fascinating book which provides the reader with an understanding of how electricity underlies all of life's basic functions and how these may be affected by electromagnetic radiation in our environment.

REFERENCES

1.   N. Werthelmer & E. Cooper. Electrical Wiring Configurations and Childhood Cancer. AmerJournal of Epidemiology vol. 109, No. 3 pp 273-284, 1979.

2.   Robert O. Becker. *Cross Currents*. (Los Angeles, CA, Jeremy P. Tarcher, Inc.) 1990.

3.   Wadsworth, C. Electromagnetic Radiation and What You Can Do to Neutralize its Harmful Effects, Townsend Letter for Doctors, Jan 1993 p. 14.

4.   Nohlgren, S. A Lethal Connection, St. Petersburg Sun Times, Sunday, Jan 10, 1993 p. 1A.

5.   Op. cit. 3 p. 199.

6.   Cleary, S. et al Glioma Proliferation Modulated in Vitro by Isothermal Radio Frequency Radiation Exposure. Radiation Research. 121, pp. 38-45, 1990.

7.   Op. cit. 4·

8.   Op. cit. 4

9.   Sutton, C., et al., Studies of Long-Term Exposure of the Porcine Brain to Radiation From Two-Way Portable Radios, Journal of Microwave Power, 17(4), 1982 pp. 280-281.

10.   Popovic P. Sutton CH., Use of Non-invasive Microwave Irradiation as a Spinal Cord Injury Model in Rats and Rabbits. Proc Soc Exper Biol Med #172. p. 132, 1983.

19

The *LifeGuide* Diet
An Optimum Plan for Human Health

"Some people have a foolish way of not minding, or pretending not to mind what they eat. For my part, I mind my belly very studiously, and very carefully; for I look upon it, that he who does not mind his belly will hardly mind anything else."

—Samuel Johnson, in
Life of Samuel Johnson
James Boswell, 1791

"The destiny of countries depends on the way they feed themselves."
—Amphelme Brillat-Savarin
Physiologie du goâut.

By now I'm sure it is obvious that the *LifeGuide* diet recommendations for a variety of health problems are remarkably similar. This is because there really is an optimum diet for the human machine. Unfortunately, western society has strayed so far from this optimum diet that we have created a number of virulent epidemics including: breast cancer, heart disease, stroke, osteoporosis, prostate cancer, colon cancer, obesity, impotence, hypertension, diabetes, arthritis, peptic ulcers and multiple sclerosis, to name a few.

Over the past one hundred years, dangerous trends have developed in the shifting American diet. Today we consume 280% more poultry, 33% more dairy products and 50% more beef than at the turn of the century. As a result, our fat and protein consumption has increased significantly, while fiber and carbohydrate consumption have decreased dramatically. The danger is compounded by the reduced nutritional value and increased toxicity of today's animal products. The key dietary recommendation for health and longevity is *reducing or eliminating your consumption of animal products.*

Patients often ask me if reducing their cigarette smoking from one pack a day to three or four cigarettes would be "good enough." Of course, I tell them that the very best advice is to stop smoking, completely. Similarly, when patients decide to reduce their consumption of red meat to only two or three days a week, or substitute chicken and fish for beef, I tell them that these are good first steps, but, the very best advice is to completely eliminate animal products from their diets. As Neil Barnard, M.D., stated in his book, *The Power of Your Plate*, "The optimal food plan, then, is a vegetarian one. Most doctors now recognize the need to reduce meat, but unfortunately, they will often dilute their recommendations if they believe their patients are unwilling to accept them. Unfortunately, halfway measures only work halfway."[1]

Vegetarianism is certainly nothing new. Some of the most influential people in the history of civilization were vegetarians including Plato, Shakespeare, Benjamin Franklin, Leonardo da Vinci, Isaac Newton, Albert Einstein, Mahatma Gandhi, Leo Tolstoy, and Albert Schweitzer.

In fact, the human body is physically designed for a vegetarian diet. Animals like cats and wolves have very short intestines, which is very appropriate, because meat putrefies when it is digested. Since the meat passes very quickly through the short digestive systems of carnivorous animals, no problem generally occurs. On the other hand, our intestines are twelve times our body length and about 4 times longer than meat-eating animals. There are other physical factors which indicates that we are basically designed to be vegetarians, including the number and shape of our teeth, our absence of claws, and the shape of our tongues.

Meat is essentially made up of two components, fat and protein. It contains no carbohydrate and no fiber. Meat and dairy products are in large part responsible for the fact that the average American diet exceeds 40% of total calories derived from fat. When discussing vegetarianism, one of the foremost concerns voiced by my patients is a fear of "not getting enough protein." Somehow we have come to view protein consumption as an imperative for strength and health. And yet, excessive protein consumption, which typifies the modern American diet, is directly linked with a variety of health problems. Although many people feel they would become weak and debilitated without eating meat, consider at the accomplishments of some vegetarian athletes:

Paavo Nurmi	20 world records in distance running, 9 Olympic medals
Henry Aaron	All-time major league home run champion.
Robert Parish	Starting center for the Boston Celtics, at age 36.
Stan Price	World record bench-press.
Andreas Cahling	Mr. International, body-building champion.
Roy Hilligan	Mr. America, body-building champion.
Ridgely Abele	8 national championships in karate, including U.S. Karate Association World Championship.
Dan Millman	World champion gymnast.
Murray Rose	World records in 400 and 1500 meter free style.
Bill Pickering	World record swimming the English Channel.[2]

Albert Einstein wrote, "It is my view that the vegetarian manner of living by its purely physical effect on the human temperament would most beneficially influence the lot of mankind." Leonardo de Vinci stated, "I have from an early age abjured the use of meat, and the time will come when men such as I will look upon the murder of animals as they now look upon the murder of men."

How much protein is enough? To determine the amount of protein you need, simply take your ideal body weight (in pounds) and divide it by three. This will give you the number of grams of protein your body needs each day. But really, it isn't necessary to keep close track of your protein consumption if your diet contains a good variety of vegetables, fruits, legumes (beans) and grains.

Beans, except for soybeans, are considered an "incomplete protein." In order to be fully utilized by the human body, they should be consumed with a grain product. Interestingly, throughout history, this has been one of the primary types of diet across the world. Even today, the mainstay in Latin America is black beans and rice or corn tortillas with beans. In the Middle East one typical meal is bulgur wheat with garbanzo beans (chick peas), or humus (a paste made from garbanzo beans) with whole wheat bread. In Asian countries soybeans and other soy products are consumed with rice.

One of my mainstay recommendations is to reduce fat consumption significantly. Of course, the easiest way to do this is to eliminate animal products. But vegetable oils should also be greatly reduced. Total fat consumption should provide approximately fifteen to twenty percent of our total calorie intake. To determine the percentage of calories derived from fats, read product label or buy a source book listing the nutritional components of various foods. I recommend *Nutritional Almanac*, by Lavon J. Dunne. (McGraw-Hill Publishing Company. New York, NY. 1990). Simply multiply the grams of fat in a

$$\frac{\text{Grams of Fat X 9}}{\text{Calories per Serving}} \text{ X } 100 = \% \text{ Calories From Fat}$$

serving by nine and divide the result by the total number of calories in each serving. Then multiply by 100.

For any particular food, this gives the percentage of calories derived from fat.

In addition to the amount of dietary fat, the type of dietary fat is critically important. Naturally occurring fats will become rancid after being exposed to the air for even a short time. To prevent this and to extend the "shelf life" of fats and oils used in food production, various techniques are used to alter their chemical structure. Perhaps the most widely used technique is simply heating the oil to high temperatures. This dramatically alters the chemical configuration of oils (which are nothing more than liquid fat), causing them to become much more stable. This is why many of today's vegetable oils can remain in the pantry month after month without refrigeration and still not go rancid. Unfortunately, when oil is heated the chemical configuration is altered to create a "trans-fatty acid," a new and completely unnatural product that has some very dangerous properties. Oils high in "trans-fatty acids" cause platelets in the blood to become more sticky, increasing the likelihood of heart attack, stroke and other circulatory problems. Trans-fatty acids disrupt the function of essential fatty acids — good fats that are crucial for maintaining the immune system, blood system and control of inflammation.

In his book, *Fats and Oils*, Udo Erasmus maintains that trans-fatty acids play a highly significant role in the development of arteriosclerosis. These fatty acids directly increase blood cholesterol and have even been linked to cancer.[3]

The main dietary source of trans-fatty acids are vegetable oils and margarines which have been "hydrogenated." Although present food-product labeling laws do not require disclosing the amount of trans-fatty acids, key words to look for when reading labels are "hydrogenated or partially hydrogenated vegetable oil." Foods containing hydrogenated or partially hydrogenated oils must be avoided. When you start reading food labels, it is amazing how often your will find partially hydrogenated oils.

For all the bad press that fat receives, it is nevertheless an absolutely essential component of the diet. Fat is nature's extremely efficient method of storing energy since fat metabolism produces over twice as much energy as metabolism of carbohydrate or protein. But, the *type* of fat is what is important. Our bodies do require fat, the *essential fatty acids*, the two most important of which are linoleic acid and linolenic acid.

Over the past century the Western diet has become significantly deficient in these essential fatty acids. Not only have we shifted to foods low in essential fatty acids, but we now consume far too much highly processed fat which competes with and displaces essential fatty acids within our bodies. The reduction of essential fatty acids in the Western diet has directly resulted in the profusion of such immune-related diseases as rheumatoid arthritis, multiple sclerosis, diabetes melitis and systemic lupus erythematosis. New research indicates that the main problem in atherosclerosis may also stem from overactivity of the immune system and may thus be a consequence of essential fatty acid deficiency.

It is no wonder that supplementing the diet with essential fatty acids is an important part of the *LifeGuide* program and is an integral part of many alternative cancer programs. Because flaxseed oil is a very rich source of both linoleic and linolenic acids (the important essential fatty acids), I recommend one tablespoon each day. In addition to being the richest natural source of linolenic acid, flaxseed oil contains natural vitamins A, E, and D, the water soluble vitamins B^1, B^2 and C, as well as many important minerals including magnesium, iron, zinc and potassium.

Although the healthful properties of fresh flaxseed oil are just now beginning to gain wide attention, its usefulness in health and healing is certainly not a new discovery. Hippocrates, in the 5th century, B.C. described the usefulness of this wonderful oil for a variety of medical problems. And as Mahatma Gandhi stated, "Whenever flax seed becomes a regular food item among the people, there will be a better health."

Always buy flaxseed oil bottled in dark containers, since exposure to light destroys its healthful properties. Check the label to be sure it was "cold pressed" within three months of purchase and always keep it refrigerated. Initially, flaxseed oil may cause some loosening of the stool, but usually this stops within one or two weeks. Within three to four weeks you will notice direct effects such as more healthful skin and hair, increased vitality and possibly some reduction of arthritic pain.

Neal Barnard, M.D., and the Physicians' Committee for Re-

sponsible Medicine should be applauded for popularizing the
new version of the "four food groups," which now includes
grains, legumes (beans), fruits, and vegetables. These four really can serve all of our nutritional needs. There is absolutely
no requirement in the human diet for dairy products, meat of
any kind, or indeed, any product derived from animal sources.
I personally believe what the Bible tells us in Genesis 1:29,

"And God said, Behold, I have given you every herb bearing seed,
which is upon the face of all the earth, and every tree in which is
the fruit of a tree yielding seed; to you it shall be for meat."

There is an ongoing debate in health literature concerning the
effectiveness and desirability of vitamin and mineral supplementation. In my opinion, supplementation is critical, for one
simple reason: Although it is possible to satisfy our needs from
food sources, foods containing sufficient amounts of vitamins
and minerals are now almost completely unavailable. The nu-
tritive value of fruits, grains, vegetables and legumes directly
reflects the soil conditions under which they are grown. Thus,
it is no wonder that most grocery store produce is profoundly
deficient in almost all vitamins and minerals. Organically
grown produce is generally higher in nutritional value and may
reduce the need for supplementation if consumed regularly.

Anti-oxidants are chemicals within our bodies that act to reduce
the damaging effects of dangerous molecules called "free-radicals."
It is thought that tissue damage from free-radicals is responsible
for a wide variety of medical ills including arthritis, Alzheimer's
Disease, Parkinsonism, strokes and cancer. This is the reason anti-
oxidants like beta carotene, vitamin E, vitamin C and selenium

are an important part of the *LifeGuide* program.

The trace element boron is critically necessary for calcium uptake and is, therefore, essential for producing and maintaining healthy bone tissue. The best sources include leafy vegetables, grains and nuts. Since a diet rich in vegetables and fruits (especially green leafy vegetables) typically supplies all the calcium needs, I typically do not recommend calcium supplementation.

The trace element chromium is required for the proper functioning of insulin and so plays in important role in the regulation of blood sugar. The chromium content of vegetables these days is extremely poor, unless they are organic. In addition to supplements, fairly good sources of chromium include brewer's yeast and whole grains.

Copper is an important element in the formation of healthy red blood cells and blood vessels. An early indication of copper deficiency is osteoporosis. Good vegetarian sources of copper include green leafy vegetables, black strap molasses, avocados, broccoli, raisins, almonds and most nuts. However, keep in mind that copper competes with vitamin C. Too much copper intake will lower vitamin C levels. Excessive craving for sugar may be an indication of copper deficiency.

Iron plays a critical role in allowing the red blood cells to carry oxygen. Absorption of iron from the diet is facilitated by B-complex vitamins, copper, manganese and vitamin A. Dark green leafy vegetables, whole grains, brewer's yeast, parsley, beets and almonds are good dietary sources. Because excess iron supplementation may actually depress immune function, I do not supplement the diets of my patients with iron unless there is *laboratory evidence* of iron deficiency.

Magnesium is a critical element in maintaining nerve and muscle tissues, as well as immune function, circulation and bone formation. Rich vegetarian sources of magnesium include apricots, bananas, brewer's yeast, black strap molasses, tofu and green leafy vegetables. Since magnesium is poorly absorbed in the presence of large amounts of fat and protein, a vegetarian diet is strongly preferred.

Manganese is a mineral which plays an important role in the enzyme that helps digest fat and protein. Like boron, copper and calcium, manganese is important for proper bone formation. It has an important role in stimulating the immune system as well as in regulating blood sugar. Good dietary sources include leafy green vegetables, nuts, seeds, seaweed and avocados.

Molybdenum, although required in only extremely small amounts, is critically important in metabolism. Dietary sources include most legumes, grains and dark green leafy vegetables.

Potassium is important in all aspects of metabolism throughout the body. It is critical in the function of muscle and nervous tissue and also helps maintain stable blood pressure. Good dietary sources include bananas, brewer's yeast, dried fruits (raisins, dates, figs and apricots), as well as avocados and brown rice.

Silicon, although required in very small amounts, is another very important element which, like copper, helps maintain healthy blood vessels throughout the body. Thus it plays an important role in preventing vascular diseases such as stroke and heart disease. It may also be important in reducing the effects of aluminum in the brain, which is directly related to Alzheimer's Disease. Foods rich in silicon include mother's milk, leafy green vegetables, whole grains, beets and alfalfa. Again, organic sources of vegetables are important since their silicon content directly reflects the soil in which they are grown.

Zinc has an important role in nourishing the immune system and in healing. Zinc is needed for properly utilizing vitamin E, and so helps reduce cardiovascular disease. A healthy prostate gland and a healthy complexion are dependent upon adequate intake of zinc. Good dietary sources of zinc include whole grains, brewer's yeast, most legumes and pumpkin and sunflower seeds.

LifeGuide
Adult Daily Dietary Supplements
Vitamins:

1. Beta carotene—25,000 units each day with the main meal.
2. Vitamin E—400 units each day with the main meal .
3. Vitamin C (ester C)—1,000 to 2,000 milligrams with morning meal.
4. Vitamin B Complex (B^1—50 mg., B^2—50 mg., B^6—100 mg., B^{12}—100 mcg., Niacinamide—100 mg., Folic Acid—100 mcg.), with morning meal.

Minerals:

1. Magnesium—400 to 600 milligrams with morning meal (amino acid chelate).
2. Copper—3 milligrams with morning meal (amino acid chelate).
3. Manganese—30 to 40 milligrams with morning meal (amino acid chelate).
4. Zinc—30 to 50 milligrams with morning meal (amino acid chelate).
5. Potassium—50 to 100 milligrams with morning meal (amino acid chelate).
6. Chromium picolinate—100 to 150 micrograms with morning meal.
7. Selenium—100 to 150 micrograms with morning meal (amino acid chelate).
8. Boron—2 to 3 milligrams with morning meal.
9. Molybdenum—25 to 50 micrograms with morning meal (amino acid chelate).
10. Vanadium—50 to 100 micrograms with morning meal (amino acid chelate).

11. Silicon—1 milligram with morning meal (amino acid chelate).

Many good multimineral supplements available at health food stores contain most of these minerals in relatively similar amounts. Each capsule of the *LifeGuide* mineral formula I distribute to patients contains the following: magnesium (AAC) 125 milligrams; copper (AAC) 1 milligram; manganese (AAC) 15 milligrams; zinc (AAC) 15 milligrams; potassium (AAC) 50 milligrams; chromium-glucose tolerance factor, 50 micrograms; selenium (AAC) 50 micrograms; boron, 1 milligram; molybdenum (AAC) 25 micrograms; vanadium (AAC) 50 micrograms; silicone (AAC) 1 milligram.

(AAC = amino acid chelate).

Again, I cannot overstress the healthful properties of fresh, cold-pressed flax seed oil. I recommend 1 tablespoon each day for adults.

Other common sense dietary recommendations include limiting sugar and salt, and completely eliminating caffeine. I emphasize reading labels to avoid hydrogenated oils, monosodium glutamate and artificial colors and dyes and other additives.

Ancient Ayurvedic wisdom teaches that digestive processes correspond with the height of the sun. This means that peak digestion is at mid-day, and that's when the largest meal of the day should be consumed. Interestingly, modern study in physiology has validated this ancient teaching.

Finally, it is critically important to recognize the importance of the mind and emotions in the digestive process. The mind should be allowed to fully participate while nourishment is being taken. That's one reason it is a good idea to close your eyes for a brief moment of prayer before starting a meal. And, while you're eating, do only that. Talking on the phone, doing business, watching television, reading a book, or arguing with your spouse, all reduce the brain's important neurochemical influence upon digestion and diminish the effectiveness of the entire process.

RESOURCES

1. *Power of Your Plate*, by Neil Barnard, M.D., is available by calling the Physicians' Committee for Responsible Medicine at (202) 686-2210. Dr. Barnard's wonderful book is an excellent "How To" resource for a vegetarian diet answering the questions people may have about adopting this lifestyle.
2. *Greene on Greens*, by Bert Greene (Workmen Publishing, New York, 1984).
3. *The Vegetarian Epicure*, by Anna Thomas (Random House, New York, 1972).
4. *Vegetarian Times Cookbook*, by the editors of Vegetarian Times (MacMillan Publishing Company, New York, 1984).
5. *The Complete Vegetarian Cuisine*, by Rose Elliott (Pantheon Books, New York, 1988).
6. *Kripalu Kitchen—A Natural Foods Cookbook and Nutritional Guide*, by JoAnn Levitt, Linda Smith and Christine Warren (Kripalu Publications, Summit Station, Pennsylvania, 1987).
7. *Yamuana's Table—Healthful Vegetarian Cuisine Inspired by the Flavors of India*, by Yamuana Devi (Penguin Books, New York, New York, 1992).
8   *The Moosewood Cookbook, The Enchanted Broccoli Forest* and *New Recipes From Moosewood Restaurant*, all available from Moosewood Cookbook Series: Berkeley, CA. Ten-Speed Press.

These books are all excellent resources for wonderful vegetarian recipes. There are many other excellent books about vegetarian cooking. The best place to get started is the book section of your local health food store.

The following organizations provide useful information about vegetarianism:

1. North American Vegetarian Society, P.O. Box 72, Dolgeville, NY 13329, Telephone: (518) 568-7970. Membership cost $12 and includes a subscription to Vegetarian Voice, a quarterly tabloid.

2. American Vegan Society, Box H, Malaga, NJ 08328, Telephone: (609) 694-2887. A $12 annual membership to AVS provides their quarterly tabloid. They also furnish a book list.

3. The Friends of Vegetarians Society (Quaker), Box 474, Beverly, MA 01915. This organization publishes the newsletter The Friendly Vegetarian.

4. Jewish Vegetarian Society, P.O. Box 1463, Baltimore, MD 21203, Telephone: (301) 752-8348.

REFERENCES

1. Barnard, Neil D., M.D. *The Power of Your Plate*. (Summertown, TN. Book Publishing Company.) 1990. p. 28.
2. Our Food, Our World: the realities of an animal-based diet. EarthSave Foundation. Santa Cruz, CA 95062. p.17.
3. Erasmus, Udo. *Fats and Oils*. (Vancouver, CA. Alive Books). 1986. p. 101.

20

Prayer and Healing
The Role of Spirituality in Health

The use of prayer in times of illness is as old as mankind. Many ancient civilizations relied heavily on the healing powers of prayer and spiritual faith in times of sickness and disease. These days, with some few exceptions, little consideration is given to the usefulness of prayer in treating diseases. Much of modern society places its complete faith in the array of highly technical procedures, devices and medicines that characterize the contemporary approach to illness.

Dr. Randolph Byrd recently completed a fascinating study at

San Francisco General Hospital, which is reported in the *Southern Medical Journal*. Conducted over a 10-month period, this study involved 393 patients in a cardiac intensive care unit suffering from various cardiac problems. The patients were randomly divided into two groups. Half received only standard medical treatment while the first names of the other patients were sent to one of several churches. The patients knew they were part of a study, but did not know which group they were in. These patients were then prayed for by people they had never met and about whom they knew nothing. In fact, those who prayed knew only the patients' first names and their diagnosis.

The results of this study are remarkable. The incidence of medical complications were significantly lower in the group of patients receiving prayer. The other group required the use of antibiotics four times more frequently, and experienced cardiopulmonary arrest and pneumonia three times more frequently than the group receiving prayer. Also the rate of congestive heart failure was 250 percent greater among those who did not receive the prayers.[1]

Many other studies have described the effectiveness of prayer. In the journal, *Medical Times*, Dr. P.J. Collipp reported the usefulness of prayer in eighteen children suffering from leukemia. His conclusion was that prayer had a significant beneficial effect on the outcome of these patients' illness.

Without question, today's advanced medical technology has given us new means to preserve life and reverse disease. But this mechanistic approach to medical problems fails to recognize the importance of spirituality in reclaiming health. In addition to reversing illness, prayer has proven to be helpful in enhancing medical procedures and speeding the recovery process following surgery or drug therapies.

And if prayer can be so effective in times of crisis, it should certainly be utilized as part of a daily program for maintaining good health.

RESOURCES

1. To obtain more information about various scientific studies designed to objectively assess the usefulness of prayer, write: Spindrift, 2407 LaJolla Dr. NW, Salem, OR 97304.

REFERENCES

1.   Byrd, R.C. Positive therapeutic effects of intercessory prayer in a coronary care unit population. Southern Medical Journal. 31 (7). July 1988. pp. 826-829.

Epilogue

The Self-Induced Illnesses of Modern Man

Evolution is an exceedingly slow but remarkably efficient process. Fortunately, environmental changes with the exception of major cataclysmic events, are also slow processes, usually measured over thousands of years. In contrast, our modern technological society has almost overnight succeeded in creating an environment which has led to a host of new ailments not suffered to any great degree by our ancestors. We are now burdened by increasing rates of most types of cancer, senile dementia of the Alzheimer's type, osteoporosis, multiple sclerosis, heart disease, arthritis, diabetes, AIDS and other problems of the immune system.

At age 15, I wrote this letter which was published in the *Miami Herald* on March 26, 1971:

> After spending three days and two nights at the Sebring car races, I found myself to be in question: Can we adapt ourselves to this future environment?
>
> Perhaps our bodies are most suited to the lush forest bed and soft, sandy beaches where former humans lived in duration.
>
> I don't believe that the two weeks in the mountains or a Saturday at the beach will be enough to keep this body, which has evol-ved under less strenuous conditions, content.
>
> Perhaps the human will change rapidly in the next centuries to adapt himself to beer cans, concrete and shattering noise. Our generations are each contributing to the evolution of pollution-resistant lungs. But what about the people of today who are stuck with the outdated machinery?"

We cannot as yet change the speed of the evolutionary process. The answer to my questions posed a quarter century ago seems clear. We must seek to create an environment, both internally and externally, which will best nourish us in body, mind and spirit. This means providing ourselves with appropriate nutrition based not on the high-priced media campaigns of the meat, dairy and processed food industries, but rather on what we inherently know is best for us. It means creating spiritual harmony within ourselves through meditation and prayer. It means recognizing dramatic changes are happening to our global environment and lighting that one candle in the darkness.

And finally, it means re-establishing a loving and supportive relationship with Mother Nature.

About the Author

David Perlmutter, M.D., a board certified practicing neurologist, is a pioneer and leading authority on preventive health care, complementary medicine and nutrition. He has gained nationwide recognition as a leader in the controversy surrounding cellular telephones and their potential link to brain tumors. He is a senior member of the American Academy of Neurology and specializes in adult and pediatric neurology as well as preventive medicine and nutritional counseling.

He received his undergraduate degree from Lafayette College where he was a McKelvey Scholar. He obtained his medical degree from the University of Miami School of Medicine, where he was awarded the prestigious Leonard G. Rowntree Award for Best Research by a Medical Student (for research in brain anatomy). He did his general surgery internship (1981-1982) at Mount Sinai Hospital and had residency training in neurosurgery and ultimately neurology at the University of Miami School of Medicine (1982-1986). He recently returned to the University of Miami to deliver the keynote address: "Disease Prevention—the Ultimate Principle of Wisdom" and "Global Health—The Role of The 21st Century Physician" at the University's Medical Student Council Convention.

Dr. Perlmutter is the founder and Medical Director of Naples Rehabilitation Center, one of the most advanced rehabilitation facilities in the nation. He is an attending physician in adult and pediatric neurology at Naples Community Hospital. In 1990 he completed training in Ayurvedic medicine.

Growing up on Florida's East Coast, Dr. Perlmutter's interest in medicine began as a child when he spent Saturdays with his father, Neurosurgeon Irwin Perlmutter, in the operating room.

In addition to his medical practice, Dr. Perlmutter is featured in both the popular weekly prime time medical television series, *LifeGuide with David Perlmutter, M.D.*, and *LifeGuide*, the national syndicated weekly radio program, both of which explore the latest medical thinking and research in nutrition and preventive health care. He authored a regular weekly newspaper column on health and nutrition, which has evolved into the *LifeGuide* book series. He has also appeared on a number of national television news programs: most recently ABC's *20/20*, NBC's *Faith Daniels* program and CNN's *Larry King Live*, discussing the cellular telephone/brain tumor controversy. His scientific research regularly appears in the world medical literature.

Dr. Perlmutter lives in Naples, Florida, with his wife, Leize and their two children, Austin and Reisha. He is currently completing the next book in the *LifeGuide* series, *LifeGuide-Vol. II.*

Dr. Perlmutter is an active member of the following organizations:

American Academy of Psychiatry and Neurology
American Medical Associaton
Florida Medical Association
Collier County Medical Association
American College of Nutrition
Board of Directors—American Holistic Medical Association
Board of Directors—Multiple Sclerosis Foundation
Physicians Committee for Responsible Medicine

Topics in Upcoming Volumes of *LifeGuide*

Acne
AIDS
Allergies
Anorexia
Anxiety
Asthma
Back Pain
Bladder Infections
Cancer
Childhood Nutrition
Chronic Candidiasis
Chronic Fatigue
  Syndrome
Constipation
Diabetes
Ear Infections
  (Childhood)
Endometriosis

Environmental Toxicity
Epilepsy
Gout
Hypoglycemia
Kidney disease
Menopause
Obesity/Weight Loss
PMS
Respiratory Diseases
Sexually Transmitted
  Diseases
Silicone Breast Implants
Skin Cancer and Sun
  Exposure
Stroke
Tooth Decay
Ulcers
Vertigo

Index

E

Ear infections 61, 64
EarthSave Foundation 14
Echinacea 165
EDTA 70, 106
Elavil® 48, 134
Electromagnetic radiation 174
Epilepsy 62
Estrogen 36
Evening primrose oil 117, 134, 137, 144

F

Fat 35, 191
Feverfew 119, 135, 165
Fiorinal® 98
Flaxseed oil 117, 133, 196
Food allergies 118
Free radicals 109

G

Gangrene 109
Garlic 38, 78, 119, 133, 165
Germanium 166
Ginger 165
Ginko biloba extract 135

H

HDL (High density lipoprotein) 76
Headache 18, 61, 127, 165
Heart Disease 105
Herbs 7, 101, 119, 134
Hip fractures 51
Hydrogenated oils 77, 195, 202
Hyperactivity 61
Hytrin® 46

I

Imitrex 136
Immune system 60, 116, 213
Impotence 75, 190